*To my father, Lim Sing, always rooting
for the underdog. I remember your lessons.*

Keeping Your Heart Healthy

DR BOON LIM

PENGUIN LIFE

AN IMPRINT OF

PENGUIN BOOKS

PENGUIN LIFE

UK | USA | Canada | Ireland | Australia
India | New Zealand | South Africa

Penguin Life is part of the Penguin Random House group of companies
whose addresses can be found at global.penguinrandomhouse.com.

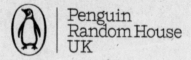

First published 2021
001

Copyright © Dr Boon Lim, 2021

The moral right of the author has been asserted

Set in 11.8/14.75 pt Garamond MT Std
Typeset by Jouve (UK), Milton Keynes
Printed and bound in Great Britain by Clays Ltd, Elcograf S.p.A.

The authorized representative in the EEA is Penguin Random House Ireland,
Morrison Chambers, 32 Nassau Street, Dublin D02 YH68

A CIP catalogue record for this book is available from the British Library

ISBN: 978-0-241-50462-8

www.greenpenguin.co.uk

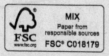

Contents

Introduction

As a Consultant Cardiologist at Imperial College London and Hammersmith Hospital, one of the largest specialist cardiac units in London, I've spent a lot of time with patients and colleagues looking for ways to improve people's heart health. Over the years I've been privileged to help tens of thousands of patients on their journey through illness and transition into health. I've devised cutting-edge methods to treat arrhythmias and syncope. In my career I've prescribed drugs, implanted pacemakers and defibrillators and performed keyhole surgeries to save people's lives. But the most fulfilling interactions for me are the ones where a patient has made lifestyle changes with life-changing results.

I've had patients with elevated blood pressure who have been able to stop taking hypertension drugs within six months of adopting effective stress-coping techniques. I've had other patients with frequent, debilitating arrhythmias completely eliminate their symptoms by changing their diet and exercise to reduce their weight, treat sleep apnoea (a sleep disorder where breathing repeatedly stops and starts) and remove the triggers of their arrhythmia. I've seen patients with broken-heart syndrome causing severe acute heart failure and have marvelled at the wonder of their full recovery within three months, having addressed the source of acute stress in their life. Patients who have reversed Type 2 diabetes through changes in their diet and exercise. Patients who have come to me describing palpitations, fatigue, skin rashes, irritable bowel symptoms or excessive sweating, who have seen all their symptoms dissipate through lifestyle measures and a shift to a positive mindset. People's ability to improve their health by committing to simple lifestyle changes is nothing short of miraculous.

So I offer this book as a guide to show you how you too can take control of your heart's health. In it, you'll learn how the heart works, what makes it struggle and what it needs in order to work optimally. The book starts by explaining what can go wrong with the heart and how certain treatments can mend it. Then it turns to what changes you can make in your lifestyle to help you keep your heart healthy and support any medical treatments that might be necessary. Together, these will give you the knowledge you need to help prevent cardiovascular issues turning into serious, life-threatening problems. For example, for many people it's a shock to learn that indulging in sugary foods on a regular basis puts their heart at risk. I will walk you through why that's the case and map out a few highly effective programmes for kicking the sugar habit.

This book can also be read alongside conversations that you, or a loved one, are having with a GP or heart specialist (cardiologist). It will help you decipher terms that you might be hearing and consider questions to ask as you discuss treatment options. It doesn't replace professional medical advice, which I urge you to seek if you think you may have a serious heart condition. I do not offer specific advice in relation to drug recommendations or surgical techniques, if that's what the condition needs, but I focus on heart conditions where lifestyle changes have the most preventive power. I have not discussed congenital diseases, heart-valve disease, heart tumours, heart infections or heart failure. For these, your specialist team will be best positioned to guide you.

As a researcher and clinician, I've taken a special interest in two areas of heart health – syncope (which is the medical term for fainting or loss of consciousness caused by low blood pressure) and arrhythmia (where, for some reason, the heart doesn't beat in a regular pattern). Over the course of a lifetime, one in every two people will experience syncope, so this is among the most common heart conditions. When people experience it on a regular basis, it can be frightening. However, as we'll see, it can also be quite manageable with lifestyle changes. Heart-rhythm disorders are less common, but can weaken a person's heart over time. This is why I have spent so much time researching what causes them and the best ways to treat them.

There are many other ways in which the heart can stop working optimally, which I'll explore in this book. Indeed, you may have picked it up because you've been told you have high blood pressure or high cholesterol, or because you've learned that you or a loved one have an increased risk of experiencing a heart attack or stroke. No matter what condition is of most interest to you, I would urge every reader to spend time getting to know how the heart works and how it is affected by lifestyle choices. Sometimes even a small change in nutrition or exercise can be transformative. This is because the heart is a complicated organ and everything we do to make its work easier can improve the way it functions.

There's also emerging evidence of a clear connection between the heart and brain, which I'll explore. This makes sense, since the heart isn't just a pump pushing blood around the body's circulatory system but also an electrical substation, full of nerves that constantly coordinate the pace of heartbeats to match the body's level of activity. And the nerves that control the heart are interlaced with ones that lead to the gut. It's no wonder that a 'gut-wrenching' emotion can trigger palpitations or that a heart attack is sometimes felt in a person's stomach. I believe that gaining a greater understanding of the heart–mind connection will have a major beneficial impact on heart health in the coming years. Already we can see how changes in our mindset can make a big difference in heart health too.

We're used to talking about the heart's work in metaphorical ways. We say the heart gives us the capacity for expressing love, gratitude and compassion. When we harness these emotions to inspire us to make positive changes in our thoughts and actions, it can be deeply beneficial for our own and others' physical well-being.

By caring for your heart and taking ownership of your heart health, you can help find your path to meaningful recovery from a number of heart diseases and prevent future problems. I hope this book will help you and your loved ones take the first step on that journey.

1. How Your Heart Works

Put most simply, the heart's role in the body is to provide a pump that does not fail. How the heart does this is quite complicated, involving not just a robust and delicately engineered muscle, but also a network of nerves that connect the heart to the brain, the gut and other parts of the body so that our blood keeps circulating without a conscious thought.

So let's start with the heart of the matter – a view of your heart's dual roles as pump and pacemaker – and how these are influenced by the parts of your nervous system that respond without your thinking.

Your heart is a finely tuned pump

As a pump, the heart is a truly impressive structure. Our bodies have about 5 litres (9 pt) of blood circulating in them. On average the human heart beats about 100,000 times a day, adding up to about three billion heartbeats over the average lifetime. With each heartbeat, a portion of the body's blood is pushed along to the lungs to pick up oxygen, and from there it travels along the blood vessels to deliver oxygen to organs and tissues, before returning to the heart to make the round trip again.

It seems obvious to us today that the heart is a pump. But it wasn't until the 1600s, when the English physician William Harvey conducted a series of experiments, that people even realized that blood *circulated* – it 'had a movement, as it were, in a circle'[1] – pumped from the heart into the arteries and returning to the heart via the veins. Fundamentally the heart does this through a choreography of muscular contractions and expansions, each timed to ensure that a manageable volume of blood can be pushed onwards to the next destination, with a loop from the heart to the lungs and another loop from the heart to the rest of the body.

In humans, the heart muscle has four main chambers that do this. There are the right and left ventricle, which together form the true pumping mechanism of the heart, and the right and left atrium (plural = atria), which together serve as the filling reservoirs of the heart – that is, where the heart receives blood back before pumping it out again. Blood goes from the right side of the heart to the lungs and from the left side of the heart to the rest of the body.

The choreography of filling and pumping is more complicated than this, involving a one-way system of pipes and gates. So let's follow the blood as it makes its journey, starting with its return from some organ, whether that's the grey matter of your brain or the skin at the very tips of your toes.

Your organs and tissues are surrounded by capillaries, the smallest blood vessels in the body, as shown on page 8. After your tissues have grabbed oxygen from the blood in the capillaries and given up carbon dioxide in exchange, the blood moves to a nearby vein, which carries it back to one of two major pipe-like veins connected to the right side of your heart. These lead directly to your **right atrium**, the filling chamber of the heart that receives blood from the body.

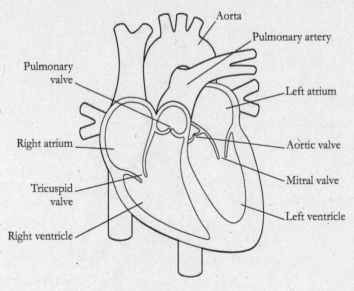

The human heart

When the muscular walls of the right atrium contract, it squeezes the blood through the tricuspid valve, which is the gateway to your **right ventricle**, the pumping chamber that supplies blood to the lungs. As its name suggests, the tricuspid valve has three cusps or leaflets. These flaps can be pushed open with enough pressure, but then they close shut, preventing blood from flowing backwards into the right atrium.

Once the blood is in the right ventricle, that contracts. This pushes the blood across the pulmonary valve into the **pulmonary artery**, which leads to your lungs.

Within the lungs, the blood passes through a series of capillaries – those smallest of the body's blood vessels. These particular capillaries are wrapped like a mesh around

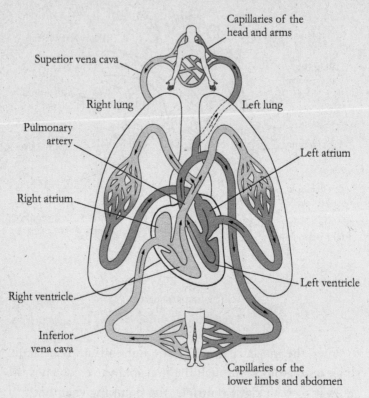

Capillaries of the head and arms

Superior vena cava

Right lung

Left lung

Pulmonary artery

Left atrium

Right atrium

Left ventricle

Right ventricle

Inferior vena cava

Capillaries of the lower limbs and abdomen

The heart and the circulatory system

the **alveoli**, microscopic air sacs that enable efficient gas exchange to occur. As blood flows through these capillaries, oxygen diffuses from the alveoli into the blood, and carbon dioxide in the blood diffuses into the alveoli. A typical pair of human lungs is packed with about 300 million alveoli, with a surface area for exchanging gases of about 70 sq. m (753 sq. ft) – laid flat, this would be equivalent in size to six car-park spaces.

After picking up oxygen in the lungs, blood returns to the left side of your heart through the pulmonary veins, arriving in your **left atrium**, the heart's other filling chamber. The left atrium muscle contracts, squeezing this blood through the mitral valve into the **left ventricle**, the strongest pumping chamber of the heart. Finally the left ventricle contracts, ejecting the blood through the aortic valve into the **aorta**, the large pipe-like vessel carrying blood full of oxygen from the heart to the rest of your body.

The blood then makes its way to your organs and other tissues along some portion of the body's 100,000km (62,000 miles) of blood vessels – a network that could wrap around the Earth's equator twice and still not be exhausted. The lacework of capillaries allows blood to flow close to organs and tissues everywhere in the body, so that oxygen can be diffused into cells to be used as fuel; and so that carbon dioxide, a waste product of metabolism expelled from the cells, can be picked up.[2] The capillaries also provide a convenient halfway station, a place for blood to be transferred from the arteries – which lead from the heart out to the body – to the veins, which bring the blood from the body back to the heart. Having made the switch, the blood then flows back to the superior and inferior vena cava, the entry point to the right atrium, completing the circuit.

The muscles of the heart (myocardia) contract sequentially, squeezing as much blood down through each valve as possible. Contracting heart muscle requires a great deal of energy, which has to be fuelled by oxygen too. Some of the first arteries to branch off from the aorta are the coronary arteries, which supply oxygenated blood to the heart itself, keeping it stoked for pumping.

But oxygen isn't the only thing that the blood delivers to your organs and other tissues. Blood carries important nutrients and molecules, such as glucose (sugar), fat, protein, immune-system defenders (white blood cells), antibodies and hormones. The relentless pumping action of the heart helps to ensure these essential supports of life arrive where and when they are needed in the body.

Clearly the heart is an impressive feat of bioengineering. But how does it set the rhythm that ensures the muscles expand and contract in the right order?

Your heart as an electrical conductor

Let's start by considering how muscles like the biceps and calves work. You have a thought – *I need to lift this shopping bag* – and you contract the muscles of your right biceps. This pulls your forearm up. Your biceps are connected to your shoulder joint with a tendon, and this contraction creates a pulley for lifting the weight of your shopping. To perform this and any other conscious movements, your brain needs to send an electrical signal (impulse) to the muscle you want moving.

But it's not the thought itself that makes your muscle move. When you think about lifting your shopping bag, the thought of this action triggers nerve cells in the brain, called **neurons**, to awaken with electrical discharges – like a switchboard lighting up to indicate a message ready to be conveyed. If a particular set of neurons in a particular part of your brain lights up in a particular pattern, it sends a signal down your spinal cord to the nerve that supplies a particular muscle: say, your right biceps. When it arrives there, the signal causes the fibres in the muscle to twitch, initiating the series of contractions that get your shopping on its way from the floor to the kitchen counter. Anything that you do consciously is under the control of the **somatic nervous system**, also known as the voluntary nervous system.

The heart is not under the control of the somatic nervous system. Heart muscles beat continuously, day and night, awake or asleep, without you ever having to think about it. In fact it would take up all your mental energy if you had to constantly 'think' to keep your heart beating – 100,000 thoughts a day for each of your heartbeats. Evolution's answer was to create the **autonomic nervous system**, which runs automatically, unlike the somatic (conscious) nervous system. The autonomic nervous system sends and receives signals to and from the heart, as well as many other organs, such as the gut and bowels, the diaphragm (the muscle that inflates and deflates the lungs) and glandular tissues such as the pancreas and sweat glands. Each of these controls automatic body functions for you – things like digestion, breathing rate, sweating, temperature regulation and, of course, your heart rate and the force of your heart's contractions.

During exercise or stress, the autonomic nervous system drives your heart to beat at a higher rate to get more oxygen, glucose, hormones and other nutrients to your cells. And during rest periods or sleep, your heart rate slows down, so that your body can recover and rejuvenate itself. In the heart there's a particular region of the right atrium called the **sinoatrial (SA) node** that receives autonomic nervous system signals. The SA node is the heart's natural pacemaker.

The electrical system of the heart only became widely understood once technology was developed to record the heartbeat in the late nineteenth century.

Devised by Dr Augustus Desiré Waller of St Mary's Hospital, London, an electrocardiogram (ECG or EKG) was first recorded in a man in May 1887.[3] In his demonstrations Waller connected a primitive version of an ECG to an electric toy train while it was moving, to show that his machine recorded actual electricity – and so electricity was what set the heart beating.

Having an ECG is a painless process. It involves attaching sensors to the skin in places where they can pick up the heart's electrical signals. Over the past century the field of electrocardiography (the study of electrical signals of the heart) has evolved, so that today doctors can analyse ECG recordings in detail to get a sense of how each chamber is contracting as the electrical charge changes in it.

Cells all have an electrical potential or charge, like a battery. Most cells in humans have a baseline negative charge, which changes rapidly as the cells receive external signals. An ECG electrode registers these changes in polarization for a specific region of the heart. When cells become less negative (depolarization), it causes muscles to contract. When they return to their more negative state (repolarization), they relax.

At the beginning of each of your heart's beat cycles, the SA node sends electrical signals to the right and left atria, the filling chambers of the heart, causing both of these chambers to contract, which pushes blood into the pumping chambers, the ventricles. This change in electrical charge is seen as a **P wave** on an ECG.

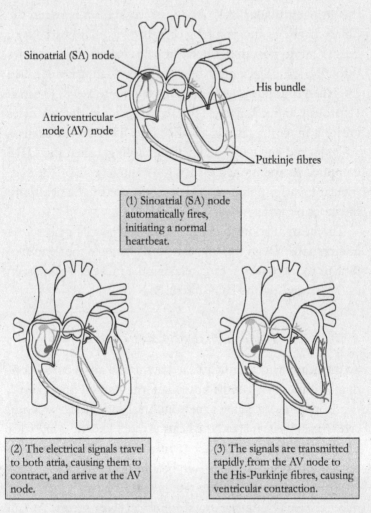

Sinoatrial (SA) node

His bundle

Atrioventricular node (AV) node

Purkinje fibres

(1) Sinoatrial (SA) node automatically fires, initiating a normal heartbeat.

(2) The electrical signals travel to both atria, causing them to contract, and arrive at the AV node.

(3) The signals are transmitted rapidly from the AV node to the His-Purkinje fibres, causing ventricular contraction.

How electricity is conducted in the heart during a normal heartbeat, leading to atrial and ventricular contraction

The electrical signal that started in the SA node travels to the **atrioventricular (AV) node**, a relay station between the filling chambers and pumping chambers of your heart. Next, the AV node transmits the electrical signal to the ventricles through a specialized mesh of rapidly conducting fibres called the **His–Purkinje system**, causing your ventricles to contract vigorously and in unison. The large muscles in the ventricles create a much larger electrical charge. This can be seen as a big, jagged spike on the ECG recording, called the **QRS complex**. As mentioned earlier, the contractions of the ventricular muscles pump blood forcefully out of the heart into the lungs or aorta.

The heart then needs to prepare itself for its next set of contractions. To do this, the electrical charge in the ventricles returns to its baseline state, relaxing the muscle. This is seen as the **T wave** on the ECG recording.

The heart is not a metronome

So the heart is both a finely tuned pump and an electrical conductor. But when people hear the term 'natural pacemaker', they sometimes imagine a metronome, beating away at a precisely fixed beat. Instead the heart is more like the conductor of an orchestra – setting the tempo and tending to be quite regular, but often varying from beat to beat.

When your resting heart rate is said to be sixty beats per minute, it isn't beating at exactly one beat every second. When you feel your pulse, you won't feel or hear a regular lubdub . . . lubdub . . . lubdub . . . lubdub . . . lubdub . . . but instead something more like lubdublubdub . . . . . lubdub . . . . . lubdub . . .

lubdublubdub. Over the course of any given minute, you'll notice that the interval between your heartbeats varies subtly, but noticeably, in a regular waxing and waning pattern, if you train yourself to listen to them.

Pulse check – sixty seconds that could save your life

Place two or three fingers of your left hand on the fleshy mound at the base of your right thumb. Move those fingers downwards towards your forearm by approximately two finger-breadths from the crease on your wrist. Press lightly and pay attention to the sensation in your fingers. What do you feel? Readjust the position of your fingers slightly towards or away from the thumb until you're confident you can feel each heartbeat.

Now focus (sometimes closing your eyes is helpful). Count how many beats you feel in sixty seconds (ideally, have someone else watching the time for you). This number is your pulse.

What does your pulse mean? Anything between sixty and one hundred beats per minute is considered entirely normal. If you're fit and athletic, or frequently do breathing exercises such as yoga or deep-breathing meditation, it can be very normal for your heart rate to be lower, around forty-five to fifty beats per minute, so there's no need to worry if that's the case.

Observe the rhythm, too. You may notice subtle differences in your heart rate, with it gradually speeding up when you breathe in or slowing down when you breathe out. This is normal. However, if you notice that your heartbeat is very erratic on a beat-to-beat basis, without any relationship to your breathing pattern, then you may have detected a rhythm disorder (see Chapter 5). It may be worth getting this checked out by your doctor.

The 'regular' irregularity of heartbeats is quite curious. Our hearts need to beat to keep us alive, and so it would appear to make more sense for the SA node – the source of all our heartbeats – to generate electrical signals with machine-like precision. Researchers wondered what would happen if this area were removed by dissection and kept alive in a Petri dish infused with oxygen and nutrients. The tissue continues to beat, but it beats with a very fixed rate – a metronomic regularity. Why then doesn't it work like that in our bodies?

Researchers tried out different things. They added a chemical called adrenaline (epinephrine), a hormone released by the autonomic nervous system in stressful situations where a 'fight-or-flight' response is called for, and the tissue started to beat more rapidly. They tried another, esmolol, which blocks this response, and the beating slowed down. Other drugs were tried too, including acetylcholine, which is released when we relax. A pattern emerged: when the fight-or-flight reflex, triggered by the **sympathetic nervous system**, was activated, the beating sped up. When the other side of the autonomic nervous system, the **parasympathetic nervous system** that controls 'rest-and-digest' functions, was activated, the beating slowed. An SA node removed from the body is no longer being controlled by the autonomic nervous system and hormones. That's why the beating becomes so regular.

Interestingly, patients who have just received heart transplants also have this kind of metronomic heartbeat. This is because when a heart is taken out of a donor and transplanted into a recipient, it's necessary to sever the heart's nerve connections to the brain – completely. Until the nerves can grow back, a process that can take several years, the donor heart is no longer under the thrall of the autonomic nervous system.[4]

The processes governed by the autonomic nervous system are regulated through the release of many hormones – not just adrenaline and acetylcholine, but also others, like cortisol, which is released when you are stressed; and insulin, which helps to regulate the amount of sugar (glucose) in your blood as you are digesting food. And although hormones are released automatically in response to your situation, you can control what situations you find yourself in far more than you may think. More powerfully, by learning to regulate your emotions and your breathing, you can improve the balance of your autonomic responses, even when you're in a difficult situation – to your heart's benefit.

As we'll see in the following chapters, some problems of the heart require the specialist tools of cardiology, from medications that lower cholesterol, to coronary stents or bypass operations to improve blood flow to the heart, through to artificial pacemaker implants that will keep the heart ticking when the SA or AV node isn't working well. In every case, changes that you make in your lifestyle – focused on the three pillars of healthy nutrition, exercise and stress reduction – can have both a preventive and a healing effect on your heart.

2. High Blood Pressure

'The seemingly healthy food that could be raising your blood pressure.' 'Social isolation during lockdown causes blood pressure to soar.' 'What can I do to lower my blood pressure immediately?' These are just a sampling of the many headlines about blood pressure that you might come across when leafing through your newspaper or searching the internet – so many, in fact, that it's enough to raise your blood pressure!

I know, from consultations with patients in my clinic, that high blood pressure (hypertension) is one of people's greatest worries. This is due in no small part to the deluge of stories about this food or that source of stress, the effects on blood pressure and the increased risk of health problems, ranging from kidney failure to heart attack. So there's good reason to focus first on maintaining healthy blood-pressure levels.

Today about one in three adults in the UK has high blood pressure. Globally, hypertension is responsible for almost 50 per cent of serious heart problems, affecting 1.4 billion people[1] and accounting for about 10.4 million deaths a year.[2] Nearly 30,000 people die each day, including 1,300 people in the US and 200 people in the UK, because of hypertension and related conditions.

So it's time to learn how blood pressure is key to your heart's health.

What is hypertension?

Your blood pressure is a measure of the amount of force that your heart uses to pump blood. As you'll remember from Chapter 1, arteries are the blood vessels that carry blood from the heart to the rest of the body. Healthy arteries are elastic and strong, with a smooth inner lining (intima), requiring less force to pump blood.

Variations in blood-pressure measurements across individuals are often due to genetic factors, which mean that your baseline blood pressure may have been inherited from your parents. However, there are behavioural and environmental factors that can increase blood pressure too, such as obesity, a high salt or alcohol intake, a sedentary lifestyle and stress. When blood pressure remains elevated, your heart muscle has to work harder to pump blood around your body. This causes more wear and tear on the heart, making it more likely to weaken.

Hypertension can also directly damage your arteries, in what doctors call 'intimal injury'. This is where small rips or tears occur within a vessel's inner lining, causing it to lose its smooth surface. Once the artery lining is damaged, fats and other substances can accumulate, permanently narrowing the arteries in places, a condition called **atherosclerosis**. This is how having hypertension increases the risk of heart attack, where blood flow to the heart muscle is blocked; or of an ischaemic stroke, where blood flow in the brain is blocked, causing damage to the affected tissue.

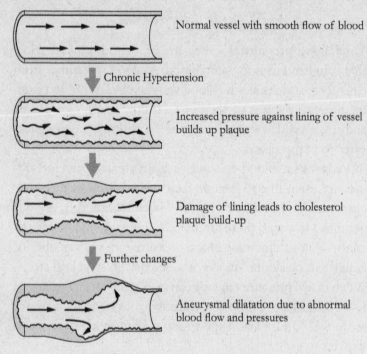

Normal vessel with smooth flow of blood

Chronic Hypertension

Increased pressure against lining of vessel builds up plaque

Damage of lining leads to cholesterol plaque build-up

Further changes

Aneurysmal dilatation due to abnormal blood flow and pressures

How high blood pressure can cause damage to the blood vessel's inner lining (intima) causing atherosclerosis

What's your blood pressure?

Hypertension is sometimes called a 'silent killer' because the symptoms don't affect people's health until a major cardio-vascular crisis like a heart attack or stroke occurs. Fortunately there are ways to monitor your blood pressure long before then. There are also changes that you can make to help keep your blood pressure in a healthier range.

Accurate, long-lasting blood-pressure measuring devices can be purchased for less than £25 (about US $40). I urge you to invest in one and learn how to operate it. I recommend starting your research at the website of the non-profit organization Stride BP (stridebp.org), which maintains a list of validated devices for use at home. You should choose a device that has an upper-arm cuff, since these give more accurate measurements. Pick one with a cuff size appropriate to the size of your arm. If you're sharing the device with others in your household, you may need to get different-sized cuffs for different people.

Blood pressure can change almost immediately in response to stress or relaxation. For example, going for a run temporarily raises your blood pressure, because the body's response to physical exertion is to increase the pace and strength of your heartbeats to supply more oxygen, sugar and other fuels to your muscles. Likewise, in an anxiety-provoking argument, your blood pressure will increase, as your stress hormones rise. Both of these spikes in blood pressure are natural and normal. Conversely, blood pressure is known to drop significantly and rapidly during relaxation exercises – within one to three minutes of doing a deep-breathing exercise like those of yoga.

To get a reliable sense of your baseline blood pressure, you'll want to take your readings when your blood pressure isn't transiently raised. This means you want to avoid taking your blood pressure in a stressful situation – for instance, don't take a reading just before you're about to give a major presentation at work. You will also want to wait about half an hour after exercising. For the best reading, you should also wait half an hour after other activities that affect blood pressure, such as eating, drinking coffee or alcohol and smoking. You should also take your blood pressure with an empty bladder – your blood-pressure reading can be up to 10 per cent higher when your bladder is full.

How to take your blood pressure at home

1. Find a quiet room. Sit down, ensuring that your back is supported, your legs are uncrossed and your feet are flat on the floor.
2. Wrap the cuff of the device around your bare upper arm, following the instructions that came with it. The bottom of the cuff should be above your elbow.
3. Rest your forearm comfortably on a surface, so that the cuff is about level with your heart.
4. Remain still. Do not talk.
5. Take three readings, each one minute apart, and use the average of the last two readings for your measurement.

What do the numbers mean?

There are two numbers to a blood-pressure reading, both measured in millimetres of mercury (mmHg). The first, higher number is your **systolic blood pressure**. This is the measure of the maximum pressure exerted by your heart during the contraction (systole) of a heartbeat. The second, lower number is your **diastolic blood pressure**, the amount of pressure in your arteries when your heart is relaxed (diastole) between heartbeats.

Whether these two numbers indicate that you have hypertension depends on where the measurement is taken.[3] If you are having your blood pressure taken in a doctor's office or hospital, the numbers may be higher, because many people find these places to be stressful. If you are taking your blood pressure at home, you may be more relaxed. So the threshold for hypertension is set a bit lower for home readings than for ones in a doctor's office. When taking an automatic blood-pressure reading, there is often a third number displayed on the monitor, which is the pulse or heart rate. This refers to the number of heartbeats there are in a minute.

Do you have hypertension?

Blood-pressure status	Home reading	Doctor's office reading
Normal	Systolic: less than 120mmHg Diastolic: less than 80mmHg	Systolic: less than 130mmHg Diastolic: less than 85mmHg
Elevated (pre-hypertension or high-normal)	Systolic: 120 to 135mmHg Diastolic: more than 80mmHg	Systolic: 130 to 139mmHg Diastolic: more than 85mmHg
Hypertension	Systolic: more than 135mmHg Diastolic: more than 85mmHg	Systolic: more than 140mmHg Diastolic: more than 90mmHg

How often should you take your BP?

More than 50 per cent of patients with a diagnosis of hypertension have other risk factors for serious heart problems, including diabetes, obesity, high cholesterol levels or behaviours such as high alcohol intake, smoking or low physical activity (a sedentary lifestyle). How often you take your blood pressure will depend on your initial reading and these risk factors.

- **Normal**: If you have a blood-pressure reading in the normal range (below 130/85 in your doctor's office) and do not have any risk factors for cardiovascular disease, then you can have your blood pressure measured every three years. However, if you have one or more risk factors for cardiovascular disease, you should have it measured once a year, even if your reading is normal.

- **Elevated**: If your blood pressure is elevated (at or above 130/85), it is worth taking twice-daily readings for two weeks. Ideally, measure your blood pressure at the same time each morning and evening, soon after waking and again at least half an hour after dinner. Record both readings in a diary to show your doctor. With this information, your doctor will be able to fully assess your risk for cardiovascular disease and discuss lifestyle changes and, where appropriate, drug treatments.

- **Very elevated**: If your blood pressure is very elevated (at or above 160/100), then take twice-daily measurements for one week and, if it remains in the hypertension range, see your doctor urgently. It's very likely you will need to have drug treatment initiated.

'White coat' hypertension

Some people find seeing a doctor or dentist a stressful experience. The natural stress of these visits can lead to elevated blood-pressure readings in the office. Up to 30 per cent of people who have high blood-pressure readings in a doctor's office have normal readings when they measure their own blood pressure at home. This is called 'white coat' hypertension, after the traditional white coats worn by doctors.

Having white-coat hypertension does not mean you shouldn't be worried about your blood-pressure reading, however. If this sort of stressful event is causing your blood pressure to spike, then other stressful events will be doing it too. If you have a lot of stress in your life, the relaxed condition in which you take your blood pressure at home might actually be the outlier – not your visit to the doctor's office!

In this case, white-coat hypertension may portend sustained hypertension and it's essential to focus on changes in your lifestyle to reduce chronic stress.

Drugs for hypertension

If you have a diagnosis of hypertension, your doctor may suggest one or more medications, alongside lifestyle changes, to help bring down your high blood pressure quickly. The drug or drugs chosen will depend on a number of factors, such as your age, blood-sugar (glucose) levels and medical history, particularly if you have a history of chest pain (angina), heart attack, stroke, rhythm disorders or if you may become pregnant while taking medication.

The recommendations for drugs to treat hypertension change regularly. Less than ten years ago, beta-blockers were commonly given. These drugs have names ending in -olol, such as bisoprolol. Today they are mostly used in people with a history of heart attack or stroke and tend to be avoided, or given only under specialist care to people with certain heart-rhythm disorders, asthma, chronic obstructive pulmonary disease (COPD) and psoriasis. They are generally avoided for people with diabetes because they can mask sudden drops in blood glucose.

The latest recommendations, at the time of writing, were published in 2020 by the International Society of Hypertension.[4] In these guidelines, three other types of drugs are preferred: angiotensin-converting enzyme inhibitors or angiotensin receptor blockers, calcium channel blockers and thiazide-like diuretics.

- **Angiotensin-converting enzyme inhibitors** (ACEs): These hypertensive drugs work by reducing levels of the hormone angiotensin in the blood. As its name suggests, angiotensin causes the blood vessels to tense up or constrict. It also causes the body to retain water and salt, which pushes up blood pressure. ACEs have names ending in -pril – for example, ramipril and perindopril.

- **Angiotensin receptor blockers** (ARBs): Similar to ACEs, this class of drugs stops the hormone angiotensin, but it does so by keeping the cells in the heart, blood vessels and kidneys from responding to it. These drugs have names ending in -sartan – candesartan, losartan and valsartan are examples.
- **Calcium channel blockers** (CCBs): These drugs prevent calcium from entering the cells of the heart muscle and arteries. The more calcium there is, the more powerful the contraction. So CCBs reduce how strongly the heart is beating and enable the blood vessels to relax and open, lowering blood pressure. Some common CCBs are amlodipine, felodipine, nifedipine, diltiazem and verapamil.
- **Thiazide-like diuretics**: Drugs such as indapamide and bendroflumethiazide decrease salt reabsorption in the body and increase urine flow (diuresis) by acting on the kidneys. This results in decreased overall fluid volume in the body, reduced blood volume in the heart and lower blood pressure.

The 2020 guidelines suggest starting with a combination of an ACE or ARB with a CCB, with both drugs at low dose, before trying two drugs together at full dose. For Black men and women, who are at higher risk of serious complications from high blood pressure, the use of an ACE or ARB with a thiazide-like diuretic may be better, depending on their medical history and age. If a two-drug combination does not bring down blood pressure, three drugs – an ACE or ARB, a CCB and a thiazide-like diuretic – may be tried.

Hypertensive treatments

This table is adapted from the International Society of Hypertension's 2020 guidelines. Drug choices must be made in light of a person's full medical history and other health factors.

Pre-hypertension	Hypertension			
	Step 1	Step 2	Step 3	Step 4
Lifestyle changes, including: Reduce salt Stop smoking Lower alcohol use Lose weight Increase exercise Reduce stress	Lifestyle changes **plus:** Low-dose angiotensin-converting enzyme inhibitor (ACE) or angiotensin receptor blocker (ARB) and low-dose calcium channel blocker (CCB)	Lifestyle changes **plus:** Full-dose angiotensin-converting enzyme inhibitor (ACE) or angiotensin receptor blocker (ARB) and full-dose calcium channel blocker (CCB)	Lifestyle changes **plus:** Full-dose angiotensin-converting enzyme inhibitor (ACE) or angiotensin receptor blocker (ARB), full-dose calcium channel blocker (CCB) and thiazide-like diuretic	Lifestyle changes **plus:** Full-dose angiotensin-converting enzyme inhibitor (ACE) or angiotensin receptor blocker (ARB), full-dose calcium channel blocker (CCB), thiazide-like diuretic and potassium-sparing diuretic

Your doctor will discuss the plan of action with you, including how your medical history influences the choice of drugs, possible side-effects and the importance of lifestyle changes, such as improving your diet, getting more physically active and reducing stress. The goal will be to lower your systolic blood pressure by 20mmHg within three months.

In those with pre-hypertension, lifestyle changes are the first and most effective line of treatment. They are usually enough to prevent your blood pressure from rising to hypertension levels.

Taking control of your blood pressure

Although much is known about the effects of hypertension, the causes of hypertension have remained elusive. Diet and exercise are well known to be important factors, although they don't explain everything. For example, Black men have higher rates of hypertension than other groups of people, and are more likely to struggle to get their blood pressure down, even after controlling for other factors, such as diet, exercise, alcohol and drug use, smoking history and socio-economic status.[5]

Other causes of hypertension may include chronic kidney disease, obstructive sleep apnoea (OBS), adrenal-gland tumours and narrowing in the aorta (coarctation), the last of which is a condition people are born with (congenital). Inflammation and immune responses are also associated with high blood pressure, but unravelling which is cause and which is effect remains an area of active study.

Regardless, you can make simple changes in diet and exercise to both reduce your chances of developing hypertension and help bring it under control.

- **Reduce salt**: Cutting the amount of salt (sodium) in your diet is the first step to take, since decreasing dietary sodium reduces blood pressure. The mechanisms of this are complex, involving higher water retention across the body and changes in the elasticity of the arteries, among other things.[6] Some people seem to be genetically pre-disposed to have their blood pressure be more sensitive to the amount of salt in their diet, though this sensitiv-ity can also be acquired. Regardless, aim for no more than one teaspoon of salt per day. This means that you should avoid regularly eating ready-meals and processed foods, which tend to contain high levels of salt.

- **Stop smoking**: There are more than 9,000 chemicals in cigarette smoke, which combine in numerous ways to assault the heart's health. For example, cigarette smoke hardens the walls of your blood vessels and makes your blood more prone to clotting.[7] Smoking both tobacco and electronic cigarettes increases inflammation in the blood vessels, and such damage can lead to higher blood pressure. Nicotine, the stimulant in tobacco often used in vaping, also increases blood pressure.[8] Quitting smoking or vaping nicotine can improve blood pressure, so I urge smokers to join a stop-smoking programme.

- **Reduce alcohol intake**: Drinking alcohol triggers pro-duction of a chemical called endothelin, which causes the blood vessels to constrict, raising blood pressure. It also increases the level of angiotensin in the blood.[9] It's best to stick to the recommendations and drink no more than fourteen units of alcohol each week, spread over at least three days; and less than that is even better if your blood pressure is high. Remember: alcohol units are calculated by multiplying drink volume (in millilitres) by alcoholic strength (ABV) and then dividing by 1,000 (volume x ABV ÷ 1,000). For example, one pint (568ml) of 5.2%-strength beer is 2.9 units of alcohol (568 x 5.2 ÷ 1000).

- **Lose weight**: Having a higher weight affects blood pressure through a variety of mechanisms, including changing the way your body responds to stress and increasing salt retention by the kidneys.[10] The goal is to try to reach and maintain a healthy weight, which is defined as having a body-mass index (BMI) of 18.5 to 24.9. BMI is your weight in kilograms divided by the square of your height in metres (kg ÷ m²). Most people find it simpler to use an online BMI calculator like the one on the NHS website (see Further Reading and Resources on page 207).
- **Perform regular exercise**: Physical activity such as brisk walking, running, cycling, swimming or high-intensity interval training (HIIT) improves the strength of your heart muscle and reduces the stiffness in your blood vessels, which, in turn, lowers your blood pressure.

Case study: Dennis

Dennis was in his early sixties and was diagnosed with hypertension. With a blood-pressure reading of 170/90, he needed to go on hypertensive drugs immediately. He thought these would be enough to get his blood pressure under control, especially because he was fit for his age – he played squash twice a week with men ten or twenty years younger than him. But I asked him to take a look at his lifestyle with me, because that was the best chance of bringing his blood pressure down into a normal range and keeping it there, long-term.

He began to see changes that he could make. He had been a smoker since his teen years and had partially weaned himself off by using nicotine gum, but he was still smoking a pack of cigarettes each week. He decided to sign up for a stop-smoking programme. He also took a hard look at how much alcohol he was drinking. He had thought a pint of bitter was one alcohol unit, but when he did the maths he realized he was often having twenty-two units of alcohol a week – well above the recommended amount. He made a commitment to eat more healthily, choosing a green salad with a simple dressing of olive oil rather than well-salted fish and chips at the local pub.

Within six months, the combination of hypertensive drugs and lifestyle changes had brought Dennis's blood pressure down to a healthy level. He was able to reduce his medications from taking full doses of two blood-pressure medications to just a single drug at the lowest dose.

Hypertension and stress

Earlier I mentioned that factors like exercise or a big argument typically increase blood pressure acutely. This is because such situations trigger the release of the hormones adrenaline and cortisol, which increase your heart rate and the strength of your heart's contractions.

Humans evolved for short bursts of stress hormones – a quick sprint away from a sabre-toothed tiger, a short struggle to overwhelm prey, a brief fight with a rival over a mate. When stressors become chronic, however, the body doesn't dial down the amount of hormones released as quickly or as entirely as it should, keeping your heart pumping faster and more strongly for a longer period of time. This is harder on your heart, which is why chronic stress may lead to hypertension and increases your risk of other heart problems.

Take, for example, the stress of being socially isolated, as many people have been during COVID-19 lockdowns. During Argentina's national lockdown from 20 March until 25 June 2020, schools and restaurants were closed and events were cancelled. Only essential workers were allowed to go to work. Everybody else had to stay home unless they were shopping for food or medicine, or getting urgent medical treatment. Because nearly everyone admitted to a hospital accident and emergency (A&E) department gets their blood pressure taken, researchers decided to see if the stress of lockdown was showing up in people's blood-pressure levels, and it was: 24 per cent of patients had high blood pressure during the spring 2020 lockdown, compared to 15 per cent in the previous three months and 17 per cent a year earlier. When they looked at people's blood pressure by age, gender, race and the medical condition bringing them to A&E, none of these variables explained the increase. The only thing they had in common was the increased stress of living during a pandemic.

Of course what exactly was causing these feelings varied from person to person. As one of the hospital doctors noted, the stress could have been triggered by fears about becoming ill with COVID-19 or financial worries about being out of work. Loss of contact with family and friends may have made stress more difficult to manage, with emotional support being less immediate or tangible. Effective stress-management tools, such as opportunities to exercise outdoors, were also curtailed. Being stressed may have led people to become sedentary and drink more alcohol.[11] All of these factors are likely to contribute to hypertension.

Chronic stress like that experienced during pandemic lockdowns is increasingly being viewed as a crucial missing piece in our understanding of the origin of hypertension. Researchers have looked at the effects of job stress and found that blood-pressure levels increase long-term, well after workers have changed jobs or been promoted, even among otherwise healthy younger people.[12] Job stress has been shown to increase the risk of hypertension in Chinese mine workers, Nigerian hospital staff, Indian bankers, Mississippi truck drivers and air-traffic controllers, as just a sample.

Outside of work, researchers have documented other links between chronic stress and hypertension. In one set of experiments, married couples were asked to engage in arguments. Predictably their blood pressure went up; surprisingly, it stayed up well after they left the lab.[13] Worrying about having money to buy food and pay bills each month pushes blood pressure up. After these worries recede, the reduction in blood pressure can last for several years.[14]

By being aware of your blood pressure and making healthier lifestyle choices with respect to diet, exercise and stress management, you can effectively manage hypertension and reduce the risks of related heart problems. These include the risk that damage to your blood vessels will attract a harmful collection of antagonists – including 'bad cholesterol', as we'll see next.

3. Bad Cholesterol

Our understanding of cholesterol is changing every year – so quickly that between the time this book goes to print and when you're reading it, new research will almost certainly be published that shifts some of what we know about the role of nutrition, exercise and genetics in people's cholesterol profile. In addition, more targeted ways to manage high cholesterol (hyperlipidaemia) are being developed for people at high risk.

For example, a few years ago researchers conducted a wide-scale screening programme of toddlers to check for genetic changes (mutations) that make people more susceptible to develop the high cholesterol levels that lead to heart disease. They found that about one in 270 toddlers had one of these changes – double the incidence previously known for inheriting cholesterol problems. They then tested the parents to identify which one had also inherited the condition, giving the parent advance warning to make significant changes to their lifestyle or, if they were at risk for other reasons, to start treatment with a drug.[1] Less than a decade ago we did not even know that many of these genetic changes affected people's cholesterol levels.

So in this chapter we'll stick to the fundamentals: what cholesterol is, what it does and the things you need to know (and ask!) if you find out that you have, or are at risk of, elevated cholesterol levels.

What is cholesterol and why do I need it?

One of the great myths about cholesterol is that it's very bad for you. In fact cholesterol serves a number of important functions in your body. For a start, it's a constituent of every cell, forming part of the outer membrane that keeps cells intact and stable. It's also involved in creating vitamin D, the hormone that keep your bones, teeth and muscles healthy; and in producing bile acids, which digest the fats you eat. Furthermore, about 80 per cent of cholesterol is produced in your liver, with only about 20 per cent coming from dietary sources. Having zero cholesterol is not what you want. It's also not possible.

With this in mind, we can get to grips with the two main classes of cholesterol that are known to be a factor in heart health.

Cholesterol travels in your blood attached to proteins called **lipoproteins**, which enable cholesterol to be used by the body. **High-density lipoprotein (HDL) cholesterol** is called 'good' cholesterol because it removes fats as well as other types of unhealthy cholesterol from your circulatory system. Having higher levels of HDL cholesterol lowers your risk of developing heart disease. The other main class of lipoproteins, **low-density lipoprotein (LDL) cholesterol**, is called 'bad' cholesterol. LDL cholesterol tends to build up, together with calcium and other substances, within the lining of arteries that have been damaged.[2]

The main types of cholesterol

Cholesterol type	What level do you want?	How can you change your level?
High-density lipoprotein (HDL)	The higher, the better	Mostly through lifestyle changes, with small increases possibly through drug treatments
Low-density lipoprotein (LDL)	The lower, the better	Can be supported by lifestyle changes, but major reductions come through drug treatments

Having more HDL cholesterol is healthier, but what's more important is the ratio of total cholesterol to the HDL cholesterol. If you have a lot of HDL cholesterol but a lot more LDL cholesterol, then the 'good' HDL is going to be overwhelmed by the 'bad' LDL.

Cholesterol, atherosclerosis and inflammation

Not many people appreciate this (doctors included!), but atherosclerosis is an **autoimmune condition**.[3] This is where your immune system attacks parts of your own body, causing inflammation.

The lining of the arteries (endothelium) is alive with all sorts of cells – nerve cells, smooth-muscle cells and connective-tissue cells (fibroblasts). These cells work together to maintain and restore the endothelium's good health. This requires constant vigilance, because our blood vessels are stressed on a minute-by-minute basis. For example, when you exercise or become anxious, your blood pressure increases, putting stress on the vessel lining. When you cut yourself, get a bruise or experience blunt compression trauma (such as clapping your hands so hard that they turn red), your vessels are physically damaged. When you go out in the cold without adequate clothing, this causes your vessels to constrict in order to focus blood flow on your body's core organs; your fingers or toes may even turn white or blue from reduced blood flow. While this is a healthy, normal response to the environment, it also puts stress on the vessels.

Although such stresses on blood vessels may last only a few seconds or minutes, the trauma calls the cells of the endothelium into action. They send out signals to attract platelets, which create blood clots; and white blood (immune) cells, which attack and disarm invaders like bacteria and viruses. Together they form a protective, healing film over the damaged area of the vessel lining.

One of the types of white blood cell that rush to the site of damage is called macrophages. These cells are the body's security guards. They descend upon and destroy problem cells and particles. Usually macrophages arrive, arrest and absorb the culprit, then move on. But when the cells of vessel linings become chronically inflamed, macrophages stick around and can cause big trouble – and when I say they *stick* around, I mean it literally.

In addition to problem cells like bacteria, macrophages like to arrest and absorb LDL cholesterol. After they pick up LDL cholesterol, the macrophages form a sticky, gooey mound, which coats and covers the vessel lining. This film does not dissipate, but instead attracts more passing macrophages and other white cells, which in turn absorb more LDL cholesterol. Eventually a super pro-inflammatory cell called a **foamy macrophage** is formed. This secretes cytokines, signalling molecules that beckon more cells to come and fight the inflammation.[4] Within this highly inflammatory milieu, LDL cholesterol is oxidized, making it more pro-inflammatory and further damaging the vessels. Although oxidized LDL cholesterol is not yet routinely measured in blood tests, it's a major player in the feedback loop of autoimmune responses through which arteries become atherosclerotic.[5]

What creates chronic inflammation in the blood vessels?

This is caused by high blood pressure, obesity, diabetes, inflammatory diseases such as lupus and rheumatoid arthritis, smoking, drinking alcohol in excess, poor nutrition, lack of exercise, stress, lack of sleep, kidney (renal) failure and . . . high cholesterol!

A localized area of inflammation and atherosclerosis can rapidly progress, with deposits (plaques) of foamy macrophages and oxidized LDL clogging up the arteries. But it may not stop there. If the underlying cause of chronic inflammation goes untreated, new plaques will form in blood vessels anywhere in the body, including those that supply blood to the brain (carotid artery), putting you at higher risk of stroke, or to the kidneys (renal arteries), leading to kidney failure. These conditions can be life-threatening.

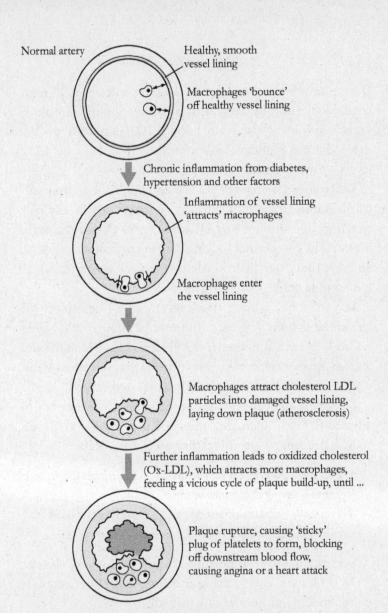

How inflammation leads to atherosclerosis

Treating bad cholesterol

If you have high levels of bad (LDL) cholesterol, lifestyle changes can help by decreasing inflammation in your blood vessels and increasing your good (HDL) cholesterol. But these changes will have only a modest effect on your LDL levels – lowering them by 8–15 per cent.

When lifestyle changes are not enough, drugs commonly called **statins** (they all have names ending in -statin) can help to reduce the amount of LDL cholesterol circulating in the blood. They work by blocking a type of protein called an enzyme that your liver needs to make cholesterol, which reduces the amount of LDL produced.

If you've had a heart attack or stroke, by definition you already have some damage to the internal lining of your arteries, and *any* level of cholesterol is likely to be too high for you. This explains why your doctor will insist that you take a statin, even if you appear to have healthy cholesterol levels.

Under the guidelines at the time of writing,[6] you also will be advised to take a statin, regardless of your cholesterol levels, to help prevent a high-risk cardiovascular event if:

- You have inherited a susceptibility to have high cholesterol (familial hypercholesterolaemia).
- You have diabetes or are deemed to be at high risk of having a heart attack or stroke in the next ten years.

Statins are also recommended if you have a very elevated LDL cholesterol – more than 4.9 millimoles per litre (mmol/L) or 190 milligrams per decilitre (mg/dL).

If you have not had a previous heart attack or stroke, and you do not have familial hypercholesterolaemia, you will probably have time to explore lifestyle changes that can improve your immune function and reduce your cholesterol levels without taking statins. Start by reviewing the inflammatory risk factors for atherosclerosis. Do you have one or more of these risk factors? If so, think about which ones you have the power to change – for example, if you are at risk for atherosclerosis because you don't get much exercise, make a plan to move more each day. If you're at risk because you smoke[7], enlist help to make this the year you stop.

Inflammatory risk factors for atherosclerosis

1. High blood pressure (hypertension)
2. Diabetes
3. Smoking
4. An inherited susceptibility to have high cholesterol levels (familial hypercholesterolaemia)
5. Obesity
6. Lack of exercise
7. Chronic high sugar intake, which can contribute to insulin resistance or diabetes
8. Stress
9. Inflammatory diseases, such as lupus and rheumatoid arthritis
10. Certain mental-health conditions, such as schizophrenia, bipolar disorder and depression, which typically increase feelings of stress.

You should also look at your risk of having a heart attack or stroke. In the next chapter you'll learn about tools like the QRISK calculator (see page 61), which you can use to find out your risk of this. A high risk of heart attack or stroke may suggest that you have inflammation of your blood vessels, even if your cholesterol levels are only modestly elevated. In this case it may be advisable to take a statin alongside lifestyle changes.

If your cholesterol is high but you don't have other risk factors, I encourage you to make changes to your lifestyle. Sure, a statin could pull down your LDL cholesterol levels, but that won't necessarily make you healthier. In fact I would much prefer a patient with risk factors who refuses a statin, despite my encouragement, but then makes a strong concerted effort to reduce lifestyle risk factors, to a patient who simply agrees to take the statin, leaves my office and has a cigarette, a double cheeseburger, chips and can of full-sugar cola. With a shift in lifestyle, you can improve your atherosclerosis risk in a matter of three to four months.

Statin side-effects

Like all drugs, statins cause some unwanted side-effects in some people. In my clinic I frequently hear the lament, 'Please don't make me take a statin – they cause so many side-effects!' Often people have read warnings that these drugs cause bad muscle aches, digestive issues or trouble remembering things. They can also increase blood-sugar (glucose) levels or cause liver problems. I get it. Nobody likes to take drugs, particularly a drug with as many possible side-effects as statins. However, researchers have shown that the pros of statins far outweigh their cons.

First, let's consider the pros. When developing a medication, manufacturers must test the drug's effectiveness by having a group of people take a placebo (an inert or sugar pill) to compare to a group taking the active drug. To be approved for use, the improvements in health observed in people given the active drug need to resoundingly beat those for people given the sugar pill. Statins have repeatedly been shown to extend the lives of people with a history of, or high risk for, heart attack or stroke compared to a placebo.

There is, however, another way that a drug can be assessed: through a **nocebo test**. This is where the side-effects reported by people taking the active drug are compared to those for people taking the placebo. Not all drugs get a nocebo test, but statins have been examined in this way. In an analysis of studies involving more than 83,000 people, almost all statin side-effects, including the dreaded muscle aches, were reported just as frequently by people given nothing more than a sugar pill as by those given a statin.[8] This study will, I hope, put your mind at ease about taking statins. The results also demonstrate the mind's power over our health. Imagine turning that power away from worrying about – and manifesting – side-effects and towards making lifestyle changes such as losing weight, stopping smoking or reducing stress!

Lifestyle changes which help to reduce inflammation of your blood vessels are essential, even if you're prescribed a statin by your doctor. Taking a statin alone is not enough to reduce your risk of a heart attack or stroke if other risks are still running rampant. A relatively high proportion of people have a second, third and even fourth heart attack *despite* taking statins religiously and getting their cholesterol levels down to levels considered healthy because of chronic inflammation.[9]

Statin alternatives

Many people trying to bring down their LDL cholesterol levels ask about natural remedies or other medicines that might be used instead of, or in addition to, statins.

Natural remedies

None of the following food-based options bring down cholesterol levels as quickly or as much as statins do, and all lack long-term evidence that taking them regularly will prevent heart attacks or strokes. However, they do appear to reduce cholesterol.

- **Plant stanols and sterols**: These are found naturally in vegetable, seed and nut oils and are sold as a dietary supplement. They have been shown to reduce cholesterol, possibly by successfully competing with cholesterol to be absorbed in the gut.[10] However, there is no robust evidence that they reduce the risk of heart attack or stroke.
- **Red yeast rice extract**: This supplement appears to lower LDL cholesterol by approximately 20 per cent,[11] but again there is no robust evidence that it reduces the risk of heart attack or stroke, or what dose is sufficient to be effective.
- **Beta-glucan fibre**: This natural fibre is found in oats, barley, yeast and mushrooms and is sold as a dietary

supplement. The fibres from oats and barley can reduce LDL cholesterol by inhibiting absorption of cholesterol in the gut.[12]

- **Nuts**: Eating certain oily nuts, such as almonds, pistachios, walnuts and cashews, can slightly lower LDL cholesterol and may increase HDL slightly.[13] A daily handful portion (30g / 1 oz) of unsalted nuts is recommended.

Other medicines

There are also drug alternatives to statins that your doctor may discuss with you, if statins are not bringing your LDL levels down as quickly as desired. They may help when taken in combination with statins.

- **Ezetimibe**: This drug, which stops the small intestine from absorbing cholesterol, usually reduces LDL cholesterol by about 20 per cent. It also appears to lower the risk of heart attack or stroke when it is taken with a statin. There is little evidence that ezetimibe has the same effect when used on its own.
- **PCSK9 inhibitors**: These are a new class of drugs that were developed after researchers noticed that people with high levels of the protein PCSK9 also tended to have high cholesterol levels. They discovered this protein breaks down the receptors on liver cells that take LDL cholesterol out of the blood so that the liver can process it. PCSK9 inhibitors stop the protein from doing this. These drugs are given by injection every two to four weeks. They have been shown to be very effective in

rapidly lowering LDL cholesterol significantly – by more than 50 per cent. They are also effective in reducing heart attack and stroke risk. However, because they are new, PCSK9 inhibitors are expensive. They are often only considered for people at very high risk of heart attack or stroke who have not seen a reduction in LDL cholesterol despite trying statins and making lifestyle changes.

If you have high LDL cholesterol, a history of serious heart problems or familial hypercholesterolaemia with other risk factors, the case for taking a statin is incredibly strong – they are tested and very effective, and side-effects linked specifically to taking these drugs occur in a minority of people. And everyone, regardless of their cholesterol risk profile, can support their heart's health by making lifestyle changes to reduce inflammation of the blood vessels. This will help to protect your heart from the worrying cardiovascular events covered in the next chapter – heart attacks.

4. Heart Attack and Chest Pain

World Cup 2006. On 4 July, Germany, the host country, was up against Italy in the semi-final match. Emotions were running high. Forty minutes in, with no goals scored, the first yellow card was handed to a German defender. Shortly after the half-time interval, another yellow card. Cortisol and adrenaline were sky-high – and not just on the field. At the end of ninety minutes neither team had scored and the match went into extra time. Fans' hearts were racing, their hands sweating. Then, at 119 minutes, the Italians scored: twice, in quick succession. The Germans' hopes were dashed. Across Germany, the risk of a man having a heart attack on this day jumped to 3.5 times more than normal.[1]

We've all heard that stress can trigger a heart attack, but when many people think of stress, they imagine stress that is related to work or financial worries – for example, a sales manager feeling the pressure to hit their month's targets, or a parent anxious if they can't pay the bills due at the month's end. But stress comes in many forms, both physical and emotional. All take a toll on the heart and blood vessels and, over time, may lead to a heart attack or angina (heart-related chest pain).

In this chapter we'll review what causes a heart attack, why you might get angina and ways to assess your risk for having a heart attack in the future. The good news is that lifestyle changes can substantially reduce your risk of heart attack, especially if you make those changes before you develop serious symptoms.

Let's begin by learning about what happens to the heart during a heart attack.

What is a heart attack?

In Chapter 1 we talked about how the heart pumps blood around the body to supply organs and tissues with oxygen, glucose (sugar), hormones and other vital elements of life. Some of your arteries lead back to your heart (coronary arteries) to provide your heart muscle (myocardium) with its own blood supply. During a heart attack some of the heart muscle becomes damaged, usually as a direct result of the full or partial obstruction of an artery supplying blood to those cells. When heart cells get less blood and insufficient oxygen, the heart muscle becomes damaged, resulting in a heart attack.

A heart attack is technically called a **myocardial infarction** (MI) – translated into plain language, this means 'heart-muscle death'. It can be scary to see it spelled out like this, but it helps to explain that once the muscle is 'dead' due to a complete obstruction of the artery, it may not be possible to bring it back to life, and the rest of the heart will have to work harder to compensate.

Symptoms of a heart attack include:

- Chest pain, often described as a central, crushing, squeezing or gripping pain akin to a tight band across the chest – this is typical

- Pain radiating to the left jaw and down the left arm
- Shortness of breath (dyspnoea)
- Light-headedness
- Sweatiness
- Nausea or indigestion
- A feeling of panic or unease with no obvious cause.

Not everyone has all of these symptoms, and not everyone feels pain in the same way. Some patients may have light – or no – symptoms during a heart attack, apart from feeling slightly 'off'. Chest pain in a heart attack is typical, but some people report mild or little pain. Women may also describe less typical symptoms, such as pain that spreads to the right arm, both arms, back or stomach. Women report chest pain less frequently than men, but this may be because they rate the pain as lower in intensity.[2] In reviewing cases of heart attack in men and women, however, some researchers think this may be more a case of women being less likely to interpret their pain as a symptom of heart attack,[3] potentially delaying when they seek medical care.[4]

> **Alert! When chest pain is a medical emergency**
> If you have an episode of chest pain that lasts longer than a few minutes and does not resolve with rest, particularly where the pain is getting worse and you are experiencing other symptoms of a heart attack, consider this a medical emergency. Get yourself to hospital as soon as possible – either by calling an ambulance or having somebody else drive you there urgently.

Some people experience early warning signs of an impending heart attack. The most obvious of these is recurring chest pain triggered by exertion or stress, which is relieved by resting. If you or a relative have this, discuss it urgently with a doctor. If the chest pain is not relieved by rest, please treat this as a medical emergency.

Being aware of heart-attack symptoms is important, because treating a heart attack early can not only save your life, but can also help to reduce the amount of heart-muscle damage you sustain. Unlike other muscles in your body, heart muscle heals very slowly or not at all. Going forward, the heart will carry physical scars from the attack. Scar tissue doesn't contract as well as muscle, so after a heart attack the heart may never return to its baseline efficiency.

Diagnosing a heart attack

There are two main tools that doctors use to see if chest pain is a sign that you're having a heart attack.

An **electrocardiogram** (ECG): Damaged heart muscle displays a characteristic pattern of ischaemic (lack of oxygen) changes in the electrical signals of each heartbeat. An ECG can indicate previous damage and can also show if a heart attack is in progress.

Blood troponin levels: Heart-muscle cells contain special protein called **troponin**, which is not found in any other type of cell. This protein helps the heart-muscle fibres contract. When heart muscle is damaged, some troponin is released into the blood. Blood tests showing higher-than-normal troponin levels suggest that a heart attack has occurred.

Sometimes other tests will be used to confirm this diagnosis. An **echocardiogram** (echo), which is a test where ultrasound waves are bounced off the body's tissues to create a moving image of them similar to the images of a developing foetus made with a sonogram, can be used to see if some of the heart muscle is not contracting and expanding as normal.

After one or more of these tests, the doctors treating you may be able to offer a diagnosis of heart attack. The hospital discharge summary sheet is unlikely to have the words 'heart attack' on it, however. Instead, it may include one of the following terms:

- **ACS (acute coronary syndrome)**: A sudden reduction in oxygen delivery to the heart. A heart attack is one type of ACS.
- **Angina (stable)**: Where you have heart-related chest pain while exerting yourself, but this resolves when you rest. This is typically an indication of coronary-artery narrowing.
- **UA (unstable angina)**: Where you have heart-related chest pain while at rest due to low oxygen delivery to parts of the heart. This is an emergency, and may portend a heart attack (STEMI or NSTEMI: see below).
- **NSTEMI (non-ST elevation myocardial infarction)**: A heart attack where the main coronary artery becomes partly blocked, sometimes in a stuttering manner. This shows up on an ECG as a depressed ST segment.
- **STEMI (ST elevation myocardial infarction)**: The most severe type of heart attack, where the main coronary

artery becomes completely blocked. This shows up on an ECG as an elevated ST segment.

Angina versus heart attack

The heart-related chest pain of angina occurs when there is a significant narrowing (stenosis) of the vessels supplying the heart, but blood is still flowing. While you're resting, the narrowed blood vessels can still deliver enough oxygen to your heart for it to pump without any problem. But when you start to exert yourself, the heart itself needs more oxygen to help support your faster heartbeat and stronger contractions, and your narrowed blood vessels cannot provide the oxygen fast enough. This creates the sensation of chest pain. So long as the heart muscle remains in a state where oxygen demand outstrips supply, angina will persist. Resting gives the heart time to recover from its oxygen starvation and the pain goes away.

A heart attack is fundamentally different from angina. In a heart attack there is usually a rupture or tear in the lining (endothelium) of an atherosclerotic plaque within a blood vessel. As noted in Chapter 3, plaques of foamy macrophages contain a range of gunk – cholesterol, other fats and calcium. When a plaque ruptures, the body's immune system goes into high gear, sending platelets to seal the tear. The platelets form a clot (thrombus). This clot may also abruptly and completely block blood flow.

When this happens in the coronary artery supplying the heart, blood flow to the heart is obstructed, the heart gets no oxygen delivered to its muscle and heart cells die – rapidly. The speed of progressive heart-muscle death gave rise to the concept of the 'golden hour' following the onset of a heart attack. During this window of time it is possible to salvage most of the heart muscle if urgent treatment to open up the artery (angioplasty) is performed.

If you have angina, are you at risk of a heart attack?

The short answer is: we don't know!

The mechanisms that lead arterial plaques to be vulnerable to ruptures, causing a heart attack, are not well understood. Researchers believe it may be related to levels of inflammation, but little is known about how to scan blood vessels for areas that are more prone to inflammation and rupture, let alone predict which stretches of vessels are at greater risk of this happening. In addition, cardiologists have found there are some people who have very narrowed arteries and recurrent angina, but do not go on to have heart attacks – they have what is called **stable fixed plaque**, a form of plaque that does not appear to rupture. At the same time there are people who have minimal or no disease in their arteries who succumb to a massive heart attack as their first-ever presentation of heart disease.

I take the view that the best way to protect your heart from heart attack is to make lifestyle changes that are likely to make any plaques in your arteries less vulnerable to rupturing. This enables you to *stabilize* existing plaques and prevent new ones from forming.

Factors that almost certainly contribute to plaques being more vulnerable to rupture include:

- **Smoking**: Cigarette smoking leads to plaque build-up in the arteries. This is just as true for occasional smokers as regular smokers. Chemicals in cigarettes are known to cause inflammation in the blood vessels and make platelets more likely to clot,[5] which increases the chance of plaque rupture causing a heart attack.

- **Poor diet**: Researchers dissected plaques from the arteries of two populations of patients – one from Portugal and the other from Sweden. The plaques in the Portuguese patients were more stable than those in the Swedish group and, based on molecular analysis, were associated with a diet with more marine-based foods, such as fish rich in omega-3 fatty acids.[6] Having a diet high in sugars can make your body resistant to the hormone insulin, which promotes inflammation and increases the chances of plaque rupture.

- **Lack of exercise and physical activity**: A study looking at the relationship between exercise and heart health over three decades of patient records found that regular exercise – enough to raise your heart rate and energy metabolism rate over your resting level – reduces the risk of heart attacks. Even people getting a lower 'dose' of exercise (for example, going on a 5-km (3-mile) run once a week – were less than half as likely to have cardiovascular disease.[7]

- **High body-mass index** (BMI): People with a BMI of 25–29.9 are classified as overweight and those with a BMI of 30 or more are classified as obese. Even among otherwise apparently healthy people who are obese, levels of arterial calcium, which cause hardening, are

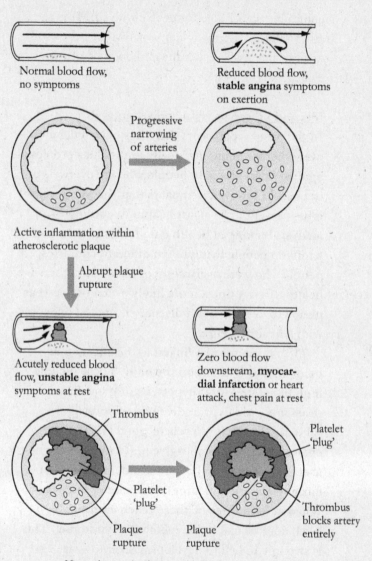

Normal blood flow, no symptoms

Reduced blood flow, **stable angina** symptoms on exertion

Progressive narrowing of arteries

Active inflammation within atherosclerotic plaque

Abrupt plaque rupture

Acutely reduced blood flow, **unstable angina** symptoms at rest

Zero blood flow downstream, **myocardial infarction** or heart attack, chest pain at rest

Thrombus

Platelet 'plug'

Platelet 'plug'

Plaque rupture

Plaque rupture

Thrombus blocks artery entirely

How plaques in the arteries lead to stable angina, unstable angina and a heart attack significantly higher than for people with a BMI in the healthy range.[8] Working to get your BMI under 25 will take time, but it will reduce the likelihood of plaques forming and rupturing.

'Fat and fit' versus 'slim and sedentary'

In the past several years there has been a debate over whether being physically fit provides protection against heart attack in people who are overweight or obese. However, it appears that shedding weight is also essential for heart health. According to an analysis looking at health data for more than half a million people living in ten different countries, people who were overweight or obese but otherwise healthy are 1.3 times more likely over a twelve-year period to develop heart disease compared to people with a healthy weight.[9]

The reason may be linked to the effects that being overweight has on the body. These include high blood pressure (hypertension); insulin resistance, which promotes high blood-sugar (glucose) levels; low levels of good (HDL) cholesterol; increased triglycerides (a form of energy used by our cells that contains a combination of fats and sugar); and larger waist circumference. When at least three of these reach a certain high level, doctors call it 'the metabolic syndrome'. This is strongly linked to developing heart disease and diabetes, but it appears that the body starts to feel the impact earlier too.

It's worth noting that the very worst outcome in the ten-country study was seen among people who were obese and had the metabolic syndrome. This population had a 2.5 times higher risk of having a cardiovascular event. But the risk was also increased among people who were a healthy weight and had the metabolic syndrome at 2.1 times higher.

So it's probably better to be slim and sedentary than fat and fit, so long as you do not have the metabolic syndrome. If you have the metabolic syndrome – and about one in three people in the UK and US over the age of fifty does[10] – then you're at increased risk of heart attack, no matter your body type or your physical activity levels.

The metabolic syndrome

Diagnosis is based on having three or more of these conditions.

Condition	What this means
High blood pressure (hypertension)	Blood-pressure reading: 130/85mmHg or higher or Taking medication for hypertension
High blood sugar (glucose)	Fasting blood-glucose level (taken more than three hours after your last meal): 5.6mmol/L (100mg/dL) or more or Non-fasting blood-glucose level: 7.8mmol/L (140mg/dL) or more or Glycated haemoglobin (HbA1c) level (a test used to diagnose diabetes): 6.5 per cent or higher

Low good (HDL) cholesterol	In men: 1.0mmol/L (40mg/dL) or lower
	In women: 1.3mmol/L (50mg/dL) or lower
High triglycerides	1.7mmol/L (150mg/dL) or higher
Waist circumference	In men: 94cm (37 in) or higher
	In women: 80cm (31 in) or higher

We've focused so far in this chapter on heart attacks and angina, but a similar process is involved in ischaemic stroke, where oxygen supply to a part of the brain is partly or completely blocked by a clot. In this case the plaque rupture either occurs in an artery in the brain or in a clot that formed elsewhere, travels there and stops the flow of blood. The actions you can take to stabilize plaques in your blood vessels will help to reduce your risk of stroke as well as heart attack.

Assessing your risk

I'm a firm believer that education and knowledge are power – the power to positively influence your health and well-being. One tool in your kit to heart health is knowing your likely risk for having a heart attack or stroke. Knowing your risk score will help inform conversations with your doctor about whether taking preventive drugs make sense in your individual case. More than that, knowing this score will be a spur to help you commit yourself to sticking to lifestyle improvements.

There are three main risk calculators for heart attacks and stroke. The main one used in the US is called the Framingham Risk Score. It is based on a study started in 1948 of people living in the town of Framingham, Massachusetts, looking at what factors caused them, and their children and grandchildren, to develop heart disease.[11] The most widely used version calculates a non-diabetic person's risk over ten years of having a heart attack based on a handful of variables: age, gender, cholesterol levels, systolic blood pressure and status as a smoker or non-smoker or person taking medicine to treat high blood pressure. Another US calculator, the Reynolds Risk Score, is specifically attuned to women aged forty-five and older. Both are available online at mdcalc.com.

I suggest using the QRISK®3 calculator at qrisk.org/three/, the ten-year risk calculator developed at the University of Nottingham that is widely used by doctors in the UK. My preference for this calculator is not merely jingoistic! I like QRISK because it enables you to include a wider range of characteristics, symptoms and conditions, so that you do not have to seek out a different calculator if, for instance, you know you have diabetes. It takes into account conditions such as migraine, lupus, bipolar disorder and kidney disease that are known to be associated with increased cardiovascular risk. It lets you note whether you have a relative who has had a heart attack, or if you have a history of irregular heartbeats, which are factors too. In addition you don't have to know your cholesterol levels to get a calculation, so you can start to see your risk profile even if you have not yet seen a doctor to get these tests done. That's not an option with either the Framingham or Reynolds Risk Scores.

I also like that you can play around with the entries to see how making a change in your life can make a big difference in your calculated risk. For example, you can input your height and weight, which together are used to calculate your BMI. After you've input your height and weight, look at how your risk would change if you dropped your weight by 10kg (22 lb), 20kg (44 lb) or more.

Most doctors would consider a 10 per cent or higher risk of having a heart attack in the next ten years to be enough to warrant targeted medical interventions in addition to lifestyle changes. If you get a result over 10 per cent, you will want to talk through your medical history, current medications and lifestyle with your doctor to identify which variables are elevating your risk.

It's important to note that scores on all three of these risk calculators are only valid if you have *not* previously had a heart attack or stroke. If you have had either, you are at very high risk of having a heart attack or stroke in the future and should be under the care of a heart specialist, who will be able to support you in making lifestyle changes alongside appropriate medical treatments.

Once you have calculated your QRISK score, please print or save it. I suggest revisiting it every six months, or any time you have a major change in health status, to see how your score has altered. As your weight, blood pressure and cholesterol levels come down through lifestyle changes, you will be able to see your risk of heart attack come down too. What a powerful thing this is to witness!

The menopause and heart-attack risk
Up until around the age of sixty-five, women develop coronary heart disease and have heart attacks at lower rates than men. This is because the reproductive hormone oestrogen helps to regulate cholesterol levels – increasing good (HDL)

cholesterol and decreasing bad (LDL) cholesterol –
and makes blood vessels more elastic. When natural
oestrogen levels drop at the menopause (on average,
around age fifty), this extra protection fades away.

The variable missing in the risk calculators: stress

Sudden stress, in all its forms, is a major trigger of both angina
and heart attack. Stress leads to an increase of the hormones
adrenaline and cortisol, which in turn cause a surge in blood
pressure, a tightening in blood vessels (vasoconstriction)
and an increase in heart rate and contraction strength. Stress
increases the heart's demand for oxygen while at the same
time reducing the flow of oxygen through vasoconstriction.

So although stress doesn't appear in any of the risk calculators, it's one of the most important things that you can focus
on to keep your heart healthy. In fact the only reason stress
is not in the calculators is because it is so difficult to measure
objectively outside a lab.

Let's consider some of the major stressors that have been
associated with the onset of angina or heart attack:

- **High-emotion events:** One of the most impressive demonstrations of emotional stress took place in that 2006
  World Cup match when Germany lost to Italy. But the
  increased risk of heart attack on the day was not limited
  to the high-stakes semi-final. On every day on which the
  German team played in the run-up to the semi-final match,
  the risk of heart attacks in the German population was 2.5
  times higher than on non-match days. Then, on the day of

Germany's third-place play-off, heart-attack risk fell back to baseline levels.[12] This landmark finding has also been seen in other high-emotion events, including on national holidays,[13] after earthquakes[14] and even on birthdays.[15]

- **Grief**: There is perhaps no event where emotions run higher than following the death of a loved one. One study found that in the first thirty days after the death of a partner, the risk of having a heart attack doubles.[16] Another study observed that about 14 per cent of people dealing with the loss of a significant loved one had a heart attack within six months of the death, with the chance of having a heart attack increased for people with a low QRISK score as well as those with a high one.[17]

- **Relationship stress**: People who've had a relation-ship break-up are more likely to have a heart attack too. Women seem to be more affected by this. In a study of people aged forty-five to sixty, women who had divorced once were 24 per cent more likely to have a heart attack; those who had divorced two or more times were 77 per cent more likely to have an attack. Men only had an increased risk of heart attack, by 30 per cent, after a second divorce.[18]

- **Sexual activity**: The heightened adrenaline drive during sex can trigger a heart attack. Getting regular physical exercise to increase overall physical fitness helps to reduce this risk.[19] Avoiding sex after either a heavy meal or alcohol (or the combination), asking your partner to take a more active role and finding positions that are less physically taxing may further reduce the chances of sex straining your heart.

- **Work stress**: Chronic stressors at work may be related to job performance or interpersonal conflict. In reviewing the health histories of more than 100,000 people in Finland, France, Sweden and the UK, researchers found that men with underlying heart disease were significantly more likely to have a heart attack when they were experiencing job stress. The increase was equivalent to the difference between being a former smoker and being a current smoker.[20] Another study observed that people under the age of sixty-five are more likely to have heart attacks on the first day of the working week.[21]

- **Waking up**: Several large studies have consistently shown that the incidence of heart attack is much higher in the morning, between 7 and 11 a.m.[22] During this period the brain and nervous system follow the body's inbuilt biological (circadian) clock and 'prepare' you for the day ahead by releasing a stream of stress hormones, increasing the number of people presenting with heart attack.

- **Overeating**: A very heavy meal can increase the risk of a heart attack, particularly in the two hours immediately after eating a high-carbohydrate feast, for example around a holiday.[23] This is more common in people who have a history of heart disease.

- **Cold exposure**: Heart attacks and angina are both more common in cold weather. This is probably because in cold weather your blood vessels constrict to preserve heat, and the heart has to work harder than usual to keep your body warm. The effect may be especially pronounced in older people[24] and during exercise.[25]

- **Infections**: The immune system's response to infection is a stress response, and so this is another common factor in promoting heart attack. In a study reviewing five years of hospital admissions for heart attack, 10 per cent had an acute infection such as pneumonia or bronchitis.[26]

- **Mental-health conditions**: A number of mental-health conditions are associated with higher rates of heart attacks. People with heart disease are more likely to have depression, bipolar disorder, schizophrenia, anxiety and post-traumatic stress disorder (PTSD), and research over the past two decades has shown that these conditions contribute to an increased risk of heart disease and heart attacks. It is not clear why this is the case, particularly since these conditions are caused by a range of underlying physiological mechanisms. Some researchers think dysfunction in the autonomic nervous system, inflammatory response or cortisol production may be involved.[27] Genetics may also play a role. If you have a mental-health condition it is especially important to seek support and treatment, as this will be good for your heart as well.

While it is helpful to be aware of possible stress triggers for angina and heart attack, the incidence of heart attacks for each of these triggers is low individually, in the order of one in a million. Watching an exciting sporting event in the cold may well triple the risk to three in a million – still long odds. So relax. Instead of worrying about whether you *might* have a heart attack while having sex or taking a walk on a cold winter's day, instead focus first on reducing your risk factors for cardiovascular disease, then on reducing the level and length of the stress reaction you have. You don't have to stop celebrating your birthday – but focus on expressing gratitude for the good things in the year gone by and on your positive expectations for an even better year to come, rather than stressing out about your age.

Medical options: drugs or a stent?

Without a doubt, if your doctor or cardiologist has suggested you take drugs, please do take them without stopping. These drugs are highly likely to help you, particularly if you have been prescribed them following a heart attack or other serious heart problem – what is called **secondary prevention** (meaning, the goal is to prevent a second event).

The most frequently prescribed drugs for preventing heart attacks are aspirin, a beta-blocker such as bisopolol (or another drug ending with -olol), an ACE-inhibitor such as ramipril (or another drug ending with -pril) and a statin for cholesterol, taken in combination. These are all well trialled and tested drugs that have a demonstrated benefit in reducing subsequent heart attacks.

In contrast, invasive medical interventions to reduce heart attacks are a matter of debate. The most common approach has been inserting a tube made of thin metal called a **stent** into the coronary artery to widen it and keep it from getting blocked again. This is done through a procedure called a **percutaneous coronary intervention** (PCI), or angioplasty with stent insertion, which involves threading a longer plastic tube (catheter) from a small 'keyhole' incision in your arm or groin up to the coronary artery. At the insertion end of the catheter there is a small deflated balloon surrounded by the stent. When the balloon gets to the problem spot, it's inflated. This pushes the atherosclerotic plaques against the artery walls, widening the channel through which blood can flow while also expanding and securing the stent in place against the vessel wall. The balloon is then deflated and the catheter removed, leaving the stent behind to hold the artery open. Because no open-heart surgery is performed, the procedure is relatively quick, with rapid recovery. It's usually performed under local anaesthetic – meaning you're only lightly sedated. However, there are risks, including but not limited to a risk of bleeding, coronary artery damage and stroke.

In an acute heart attack where the coronary artery is completely blocked, PCI is highly appropriate. Putting in a stent will relieve severe chest symptoms immediately and can save the person's life. What is less clear is the benefit of using PCI in people who are experiencing recurrent but stable angina.

For decades, many patients with angina were given stents as the 'gold standard' preventive measure against heart attack. But in 2017 Professor Darrel Francis from Imperial College London and his colleagues shook up the field of cardiology when they published a study of stenting for angina in the medical journal *The Lancet*.[28] In the study, called ORBITA, a group of patients with symptoms of reduced blood supply to the tissues was recruited. All were given six weeks of medication. Then half were randomly assigned to have a PCI and get a stent, while the other half were randomly assigned to have a sham procedure. This was the first time stenting was compared to something that looked like stenting to the patient. The people going through the sham procedure were hooked up to heart monitors, a catheter was inserted through a keyhole incision and the catheter was then threaded up to the coronary artery. However, at that point the balloon was not inflated and no stent was put in place. None of the patients knew which procedure they had had, nor did the clinical staff who escorted them to recovery or watched over them there. Even the researchers who conducted follow-up examinations of the patients six weeks later were in the dark about which procedure each person had gone through. The ORBITA study was a model trial: randomized (participants were randomly assigned to get treatment or the sham), double-blinded (neither the participants nor the researchers knew which treatment the participants received while the study was happening) and sham-controlled (the treatment and the sham seemed exactly the same to the participants).

As you've no doubt already worked out, both groups of patients saw similar improvements in sustained exercise time and reduction in angina symptoms after their procedure. In other words, the people who got the sham fared just as well as those who had a stent put in place. Stenting did not add any preventive benefit.

People – both patients and doctors – are often eager to have immediate fixes for conditions, particularly ones like recurring angina that can signal that an acute heart attack may be lurking in the future. It is tempting to think we can put a stent in a coronary artery and reduce this threat. But if you have plaques building up in arteries throughout your body, which is the case in about 50 per cent of patients, then putting a stent in the coronary artery is not going to keep plaques elsewhere from rupturing.

To keep your heart healthy, you need to take a holistic approach – reducing hypertension, reducing cholesterol, stopping smoking, reducing strain on the heart through losing weight and improving the tone of heart muscle through regular exercise. These interventions take time and commitment, but when you keep to them, they are incredibly effective in reducing your cardiovascular risk.

Preventing heart attacks

More than 95 per cent of the population who are 'heart well' – people who have not had a major cardiovascular event, many of whom have no other known health issue – aren't focusing on the things they can do to keep their heart healthy right now. All too often, people take for granted that they are healthy until their body sends up a red alert that they're not. Unfortunately it can take ten to twenty, or even thirty, years of bad lifestyle choices to bear fruit in the form of recurring angina or a heart attack. By then it's harder to undo years of habit and your arteries may be permanently narrowed.

By picking up this book you've decided to take care of your heart – not next year or next month, but *right now*. Perhaps you've been diagnosed with a serious heart problem and you're looking for the motivation to build new habits. That's great. Perhaps you did it because a friend or family member has had a heart attack and you wanted to support them. Let this be a jolting wake-up call for you too. Or perhaps you have a stressful job and home situation and have read stories about how this can trigger a heart attack.

Whatever got you to this moment, seize the opportunity to commit yourself to lifestyle changes that will help reduce the risk to your heart.

5. Rhythm Disorders

I vividly remember the very first time I made a heart stop beating.

I was in the middle of my PhD studies at Imperial College London, pushing heavy trolleys of electrical recording and stimulating equipment into surgical theatres to find and stimulate the nerve cells hiding around the heart to see how they might reveal a solution to each patient's medical condition. On this day I'd placed an electrode just outside the heart of a person undergoing open-chest surgery and, at the lead surgeon's cue, turned on the electrical current. And then it happened – the heart just stopped. The electrocardiogram (ECG) monitor was a flat line, six seconds without any electrical activity from the heart at all. Seven seconds. Eight. I felt my own heart starting to race, panicked. Then the surgeon smiled at me, nonchalantly picked up a pair of forceps (surgical tongs) and started tapping on the inert heart muscle, like a world-class percussionist striking the head of a timpani drum. This tapping spurred the muscle to contract, setting the heart back to beating.

The experience taught me a lot about the autonomic nervous system: how to find and stimulate the heart's nerves, how these nerves cause the heart's filling chambers to beat abnormally and, most importantly, why it's important to remain cool and collected in any emergency situation, in and out of a surgical theatre. My knowledge of the heart's nerve cells has also grown hugely since my student days and, with many years of experience as a clinician and researcher, I've been able to pioneer new techniques for rhythm disorders (arrhythmias) that take advantage of the role of the autonomic nervous system, including the UK's first successful procedure to stimulate and stop the electrical signals in a complex of nerves (plexus) connected to a person's pulmonary veins. This set of nerves had been causing one of my patients to experience debilitating episodes of arrhythmia. The procedure has fixed her arrhythmias, permanently.[1]

Many things can make a heart miss or skip beats, and having an arrhythmia puts more strain on your heart. Thankfully, once you become aware of a rhythm disorder, there are many things you can do to help keep your heart in good stead, whether or not your heart needs a nudge to get it back 'on beat'.

How do heartbeats get 'disordered'?

I mentioned in Chapter 1 that the heart is not a metronome. If the heart does not beat regularly when it is beating normally, you may be wondering what exactly counts as a rhythm disorder.

Generally, heart-rhythm disorders are clustered in two groups:

- **Tachycardia**, or rapid heartbeats – faster than 100 beats per minute
- **Bradycardia**, or slow heartbeats – slower than 60 beats per minute.

Both of these arrhythmias can lead to **palpitations**, which is a way of describing any abnormal heart rhythm you notice. Some people report that they feel as though their heart is pounding in their chest like it's going to pop out. Others say they feel a fluttering or flip-flopping. Often there's a sense that the heart is racing, but unevenly – speeding up and slowing down, out of step with what they're doing. They may sense their heartbeat in their throat or neck, and not just in their chest.

Palpitations are a symptom, not a diagnosis, however. If you have two double espressos, then find yourself rushing around to get to your next important meeting, you may well experience palpitations. This does not necessarily mean that you have an arrhythmia.

> **Alert! When you experience _more_ than palpitations**
> With some abnormal rhythms, people feel symptoms other than palpitations. These include dizziness, chest pain, shortness of breath and collapses with loss of consciousness. If you experience any of these symptoms, please speak to your doctor urgently.

A normal heartbeat is called **normal sinus rhythm**. As you may remember from Chapter 1, this is where cells in the sinoatrial (SA) node become less negative in electrical charge (depolarize), causing the muscles of the heart's top two filling chambers (atria) to contract. This change is picked up by the electrodes in an ECG and is recorded as the P wave. Within two-tenths of a second, the electrical impulse that originated in the SA node is relayed to the atrioventricular (AV) node, and then it's transmitted through the network of tissue called the His–Purkinje system. This rapid conduction of electricity causes the muscles of the heart's two pumping chambers (ventricles) to contract. These changes show up on an ECG as the QRS complex. Finally, when the ventricles relax, it shows up as the T wave. Then, if everything is working correctly, it all starts again.

You have a rhythm disorder if your heartbeat doesn't always follow the normal sinus pattern. This can happen in a variety of ways. For example, electrical signals might arise in two places, creating 'competing' heartbeats, or electricity might flow almost continuously without pauses, so that the chambers don't get time to relax fully.

The symptoms of different arrhythmias may be felt in different ways. But take a moment to review the table overleaf and appreciate something common to almost all heart-rhythm disorders: you may have *no symptoms at all*. Because some people

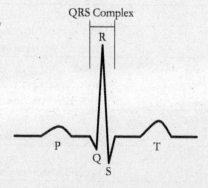

The electrical signal of normal (sinus) rhythm

with an arrhythmia may never experience palpitations, they may not realize they have a condition until the strain on their heart causes other symptoms, such as shortness of breath or fatigue.

Types of arrhythmia and how they relate to palpitations

Rhythm	Types of palpitations typically reported
Normal sinus rhythm	None
Sinus bradycardia (rhythm less than 60bpm)	None Slow, strong beats
Sinus tachycardia (rhythm more than 100bpm)	None Racing beats
Atrial or supraventricular ectopy or ectopic beats (SVE); also called premature atrial complex (PAC)	None Extra, skipped, strong, lurching, rapid beats 'Fluttering' in the chest
Ventricular ectopy or ectopic beats (VE), also called premature ventricular complex (PVC)	None Extra, skipped, strong, lurching, rapid beats 'Fluttering' in chest
Atrial fibrillation (AF or AFib)	None Chaotic, rapid, irregular, 'flip-flopping', pounding beats
Supraventricular tachycardia (SVT)	None Sudden-onset, rapid, regular beats, sometimes with the neck pounding
Ventricular tachycardia (VT)	None Rapid, regular, pounding beats
Heart block (first degree, second degree or third degree)	None Skipped, slow, strong beats

Ectopic heartbeats

The relentless firing of electrical impulses in the SA node is tightly regulated by the autonomic nervous system. Some rhythm disorders are caused by electrical impulses originating from somewhere other than the SA node. This is called **ectopy**, taken from the Greek word *ektopos*, meaning 'foreign' or 'away from a place'.

In an ectopic heartbeat, nerve cells outside the SA node fire intermittently, making parts of the heart muscle contract out of time with the SA node's impulses. This causes the SA node to temporarily stop sending impulses, with pauses typically lasting two to three seconds.

Ectopic beats can arise in either of the atria or the ventricles. They are very common. Having up to 500 ectopic beats over a twenty-four-hour period – about 0.5 per cent of the average 100,000 heartbeats that a human has per day – is considered normal. Some ectopic beats can be exaggerated by stress or illness. These usually resolve after a few weeks or months.

It's possible to pinpoint where the extra beats are originating using an ECG. However, people who have ectopic beats may not get them so regularly that they will show up during an appointment with a heart specialist, or even during a visit to A&E following a particularly upsetting episode of palpitations or other symptoms. For this reason, if you have infrequent ectopic beats, you may want or be asked to use a mobile ECG recording device. Personal devices like the Apple Watch Series 4 or higher, or an AliveCor KardiaMobile ECG, which can be paired with an iPhone and many Android phones and tablets, provide accurate recordings. These can be used during less frequent episodes of ectopic beats. Or your heart specialist may provide you with a single-lead portable ECG device.

If you decide to invest in a personal mobile device, it is usually quick to set up – it takes under two minutes. It can record continuous ECG traces of ectopic beats for thirty to sixty seconds at a time, but it can sometimes be difficult to get a recording started before a short-lived episode has ended. If you do manage to capture a recording like this, please download the data to show your doctor. Such recordings are extremely helpful – and instead of having to wait for a second consultation, your cardiologist may be able to make a clear diagnosis at your first meeting and get you started on treatment sooner. (To see videos of these devices recording ectopic beats, visit drboonlim.co.uk/heart-healthy.)

Most patients who experience ectopic beats feel the delayed sinus beat that follows the ectopic beat rather than the ectopic beat itself. This is because when the SA node pauses, the ventricles are given more time to fill up, so a stronger contraction

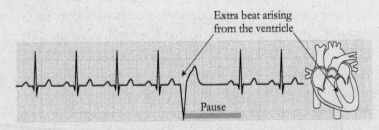

Extra beat arising from the ventricle

Pause

An ectopic beat arising from the ventricle (pumping chamber) – the extra, broad beat is indicated by the arrow, which is followed by a pause in the regular heartbeat, indicated by the bar

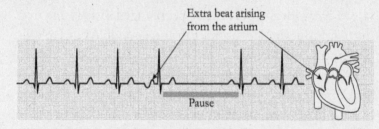

An ectopic beat in an atrium (filling chamber) – the extra beat is
indicated by the arrow, which is followed by a pause in the
regular heartbeat, indicated by the bar

of the ventricles is needed to push all the blood out of the
heart. The experience can be extremely disconcerting. I've
had patients say it feels as if their heart is 'jumping out of the
chest', 'lurching' or 'stopping me in my tracks'. Some patients
feel pain.

Having ectopic beats can set off a feedback loop of worry
and anxiety, where concern that there is something wrong
with the heart leads to stress and an acute rise in adrenaline,
which then provokes even more ectopics and more stress. If
you have ectopic beats somewhat infrequently and your doctor examines you and everything else appears normal, rest
easy: your symptoms are probably nothing to worry about.
Knowing this might be enough to break the cycle and improve
your overall feeling of well-being.

Atrial fibrillation

The most common arrhythmia is **atrial fibrillation** (AF), often
called AFib for short. The chances of having AFib increase

as we age, with 4–5 per cent of people aged seventy and over having it. But younger people can also develop AFib, typically in response to triggers.

When you are diagnosed with AFib, it means there's an abnormality in your heart rhythm where the atria beat out of sync, creating chaotic electrical heart signals. These chaotic signals kick the ventricles out of beat too, making your heartbeat irregular. During AFib the chaos of electrical signals often sets the heart racing. You may see your pulse rate jump up to 100–175 beats per minute (tachycardia), compared to the normal pulse of 60–100 beats per minute.

In addition, the pulse's irregularity is often great enough to be felt and seen. If you feel your heart racing unexpectedly, try doing the pulse check (see page 15). If this is happening regularly, you may want to use the KardiaMobile ECG, Apple Watch or a device provided by your doctor or cardiologist to record your heartbeat.

It may seem as though having an irregular heartbeat every now and then isn't something to be too concerned about. However, frequent episodes of rapid irregular heartbeats can significantly compromise your health. Imagine asking your heart to run a marathon twenty-four hours a day, sustaining a pulse in excess of 100 beats per minute – this is akin to the demands that AFib puts on your heart. The heart can tire and weaken without rest, leading it to fail. AFib also increases by up to fivefold the risk of having a stroke and, when a stroke occurs, it is more likely to have serious disability afterwards.[2] With appropriate treatment, AFib can be controlled or reversed, putting you at much less risk of these potentially life-threatening conditions.

For these reasons it's important to be aware of the symptoms of AFib and to seek treatment if you think you have it. With AFib, you may experience:

- Palpitations, the odd sensation of irregular, weak and strong heartbeats, which may feel like a flip-flopping, racing or uncomfortable sensation in the chest
- Chest pain (angina)
- Light-headedness or dizziness
- A constant feeling of tiredness or weakness that is not relieved by regular sleeping (fatigue)
- Weakness
- Inability to exercise
- Shortness of breath (dyspnoea).

Other arrhythmias

Although ectopic beats and AFib are the most common, there are several other types of heart-rhythm disorders, including atrial flutter, supraventricular tachycardia (SVT), premature ventricular contractions (PVC), ventricular tachycardia (VT), sick-sinus syndrome and heart block. In one type of supraventricular tachycardia, called Wolff-Parkinson-White (WPW) syndrome, people are born with an extra electrical pathway between the atria and the ventricles, creating the potential for a continuous electrical circuit in the heart that causes sudden, rapid palpitations.

Deciphering rhythm disorders

The names of these conditions may sound confusing, but if you crack the code of medical jargon, you can often work out what they involve:

- **Fibrillation:** chaotic electrical signals
- **Atrial:** the disorder starts in one of the heart's filling chambers (atria)
- **Ventricular:** the disorder starts in one of the heart's pumping chambers (ventricles)
- **Supraventricular:** the disorder starts above (supra) the ventricles, in the atria
- **Sinus:** another term for the SA node, the heart's pacemaker; when it's 'sick', the pulse can vacillate between fast (tachycardia) and slow (bradycardia)
- **Heart block:** a delay or pause in how electrical signals travel from an atrium to a ventricle
- **Tachycardia:** rapid heartbeats, faster than 100 beats per minute
- **Bradycardia:** slow heartbeats, slower than 60 beats per minute.

Some rhythm disorders appear to be genetic, passed down from generation to generation. Common inherited arrhythmias include Brugada syndrome, long QT syndrome and short QT syndrome. Some studies suggest that atrial fibrillation may also be inherited.[3] Just as with non-inherited rhythm disorders, people with inherited arrhythmias may experience symptoms of palpitations, dizziness, blackouts or shortness of breath.

Unfortunately, for some families the first sign of an abnormality is when someone dies suddenly, without any obvious cause, particularly if the person is under the age of sixty. If you have a first-degree relative – a parent, sibling or child – who has been diagnosed with an inherited arrhythmia, it's recommended that you are referred to a cardiologist with an interest in inherited conditions, to consider onward management, including possible genetic testing.

Diagnosing heart-rhythm disorders

If you have an irregular heartbeat, your doctor will review your medical history and conduct a thorough physical examination. You might be asked to undergo the following tests:

- **Electrocardiogram** (ECG): The primary tool for diagnosing heartbeat problems because it shows the rhythm of contractions and relaxations of each of the heart's chambers. However, clinic ECGs may not be helpful for recording rhythm disorders that happen intermittently, since you won't always be in the clinic when they occur.
- **Holter monitor**: This is a portable continuous ECG recording device that is stuck to your chest using adhesive patches. You'll be asked to wear it for one to fourteen days, pressing a button to annotate each time you feel your heartbeat becoming irregular or fast.
- **Echocardiogram** (echo): A non-invasive test that uses ultrasound waves to create images of the heart and its underlying structures in motion. It can be used to rule out problems with your heart muscle or valves.

- **Exercise stress test**: This involves recording an ECG while you're running on a treadmill or riding an exercise bicycle to see if physical exertion triggers a rhythm disorder.
- **Blood tests**: These can be used to rule out abnormal blood-count levels, thyroid problems or heart-muscle dysfunction.

What triggers arrhythmia?

In more than two-thirds of people, rhythm disorders are triggered by the autonomic nervous system, the part of the nervous system that governs that host of day-to-day bodily functions that we don't think about or consciously control.[4] Among other things, the autonomic nervous system controls how our body reacts to stress and how it operates during rest and digestion – two common triggers for arrhythmia.

Stress: The sympathetic nervous system governs the fight-or-flight reflex, which allows you to run for your life, or fight for it, without giving it a second thought. A major component of this response is the release of the hormones adrenaline and cortisol, which speeds up the heart rate to get more fuel delivered to your muscles, to ensure they are ready for action. Many people with rhythm disorders can recall stress triggering an episode. The culprit can be 'invited' stress, such as getting exercise or drinking a cup of coffee or alcohol, or less welcome stress, such as a big deadline at work. Arrhythmia can also be triggered by an infection, which the body meets with both an immune response and a heightened stress response.

Sleep and digestion: The flipside of this is the rest-and-digest mode, when the parasympathetic nervous system settles you into a deeply relaxed state to allow your body time to convert food into energy and rejuvenate itself during sleep. This involves quieting or slowing several bodily functions, including the heart and breathing rate. The vagus nerve – the main complex of nerves that govern the parasympathetic nervous system – runs from the brain to the heart and lungs and down to the gut, intimately connecting these organs.

Think of the vagus as a large motorway full of cars travelling in two directions, from the brain to the gut and from the gut to the brain. Along the way there's a junction – the heart – where cars can turn off, if traffic gets too heavy. When a certain level of electrical traffic spills over into the heart, it can trigger heart-rhythm abnormalities such as ectopic beats and AFib.

You may not realize that electrical signals are travelling in both directions, but they are. When you eat a sizeable amount of food, the linings of your oesophagus, stomach and other intestinal organs stretch, and this stretching activates the vagus nerve. Sensory nerves carry signals, such as the feeling of being full, up from the gut to the brain; and in response motor fibres carry signals, such as the command to make different parts of the gut contract one after the other during digestion (peristalsis), down from the brain to the gut. Some of this electrical activity stimulates the heart's nerves.

Most of the patients in my clinic who have ectopic beats or AFib can recall episodes during or soon after eating a large meal, drinking alcohol, feeling bloated, burping or having acute stomach cramp or lower abdominal pain. Equally, when

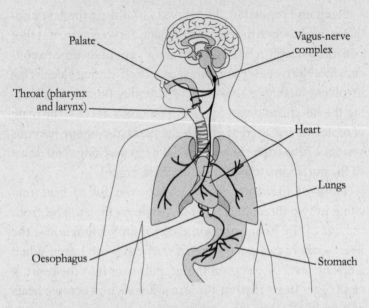

Palate

Vagus-nerve
complex

Throat (pharynx
and larynx)

Heart

Lungs

Oesophagus

Stomach

The gut-heart-brain connection helps explain why some rhythm disorders are triggered by abdominal symptoms such as bloating and cramp. The autonomic nervous-system fibres run between the brain and gut. Electrical nerve signals travel in both directions along the nerve fibres and can spill over into the heart's nerves, triggering arrhythmia.

people have frequent episodes of ectopic beats in a repeating pattern, some of them find that releasing stomach gas with a burp improves their symptoms.

When you're sleeping, the parasympathetic system is also sending signals along the vagus nerve to slow your breathing and heart rate and to quieten your motor system. If there has been a particularly strong parasympathetic trigger – for example, doing a hard physical workout or eating a large meal in the preceding hours – then the surge in vagus-nerve activity may trigger AFib, causing you to wake abruptly from your sleep with palpitations. This form of AFib, called **vagally mediated AFib,** is more commonly seen in younger people, aged about thirty to fifty.

You may be able to get irregular heartbeats under control by understanding your triggers and avoiding them. Avoiding big meals, excessive amounts of caffeine, alcohol binges or heavy workouts, or reducing stress, can improve symptoms. Keeping a diary will help you become more aware of triggers.

The connection between sleep disorders and rhythm disorders

Some episodes of arrhythmia during sleep are not triggered by rest, but by stress. This is the case in people with **obstructive sleep apnoea** (OSA), a disorder where the airway gets temporarily blocked during sleep, causing them to experience pauses in their breathing. The lack of air jerks the sympathetic nervous system into action, startling them awake as they gasp for air before falling back into slumber.

This may not sound like anything you have experienced, but some people with sleep apnoea are not aware it's happening to them, because they don't fully wake up from sleep when their body gasps for air. For these individuals, the most noticeable symptom may be excessive sleepiness or fatigue during waking hours, or regularly waking up with a headache in the morning. Another sign is heavy snoring, which might be loud enough to wake a partner or family member, but not the sleeper. It's worth asking your sleeping partner or others in your household if you snore.

Sleep apnoea initiates AFib and other arrhythmias by triggering the body's stress response, often many times each night. Imagine that you are crossing the road, turn your head and suddenly see a juggernaut barrelling right towards you. That would get your heart racing and take your breath away, right? And your autonomic nervous system would be right to release that huge surge of adrenaline and cortisol, because it might just be enough to get you out of the way of the truck. But as soon as you get yourself to safety, you decide to try and cross the road again, turn your head and suddenly see a juggernaut barrelling right towards you. Your heart would start racing again. You get yourself to safety, try to cross again – another juggernaut. That's the sort of stress your heart is enduring during a night punctuated by episodes of sleep apnoea. Coming out of the slow heart and breathing rate of sleep, these repeated jolts of low oxygen and high adrenaline and cortisol trigger arrhythmia, most commonly AFib.

There are also clear links between sleep apnoea and other heart problems. It's possible that the constant fluctuations in blood oxygen levels caused by sleep apnoea contribute to inflammation of the arteries, obstruction of blood flow, insulin resistance and high blood pressure.

People who are overweight or obese are at higher risk of having obstructive sleep apnoea because a larger chest and neck size increase the likelihood of airway compression. Sleep apnoea may happen more frequently when sleeping flat on your back, and during REM sleep when your muscles are more relaxed.

If you snore, are overweight or obese, have diabetes or hypertension, you should ask your doctor about getting screened for sleep apnoea. The main way to treat sleep apnoea is to lose weight, but a night mask providing continuous positive airway pressure (CPAP) can be very helpful and can reduce arrhythmia symptoms too.

Treating atrial fibrillation and other arrhythmias

Having AFib increases your risk of stroke, and your doctor will assess this risk and prescribe anticoagulation medication (which helps prevent blood clots), if necessary, to reduce this risk. However, the principal goal in treating AFib and other rhythm abnormalities is to reset the heart's rhythm. Given that nearly all of these conditions are triggered by the autonomic nervous system, choosing to make lifestyle changes – including avoiding stress – can significantly improve the frequency of your episodes and your symptoms.

Other drugs may be prescribed where lifestyle interventions fail to make sufficient difference. If you don't seem to have any symptoms other than a racing heart, then a reasonable strategy is to maintain a healthy heart rate (below 100 beats per minute) by taking a rate-control drug such as a beta-blocker or calcium channel blocker, the most commonly prescribed drugs for heart-rhythm abnormalities.

Beta-blockers: These drugs block the hormone adrenaline from attaching to receptors on the cells of the heart, slowing the heart rate down, reducing the strength of contractions and thus reducing the risk of developing arrhythmia. These drugs have names ending in -lol, such as bisoprolol, metoprolol or carvedilol.

Calcium channel blockers (CCBs): These drugs, including diltiazem and verapamil, prevent calcium from entering the cells of the heart muscle. Because excessive calcium within the heart's cells can lead to ectopic beats, reducing calcium helps regulate the heartbeat.

Your doctor will be able to discuss these and other drug options further with you, to help you understand the advantages and disadvantages of each. Where lifestyle changes and drugs are not working to reduce episodes, there are other options that may reset your heart's rhythm back to normal.

Electrical cardioversion: This is where an electrical shock (impulse) is delivered to the heart to reset its rhythm. Electrode pads are placed on the chest and a calibrated electric current is delivered to stop the arrhythmia. You are put under general anaesthesia for this.

Catheter ablation: For this, your heart specialist (electrophysiologist) identifies specific areas in the heart that appear to be giving rise to abnormal electrical signals and either freezes (cryoablation) or burns (radiofrequency ablation) the tissue.[5] This creates scar tissue that stops the abnormal signals from occurring. The ablation is delivered by threading electrical wires from a keyhole incision in the groin to the heart. These approaches have improved tremendously over the past several years, with ablation curing more than 95 per cent of atrial flutter, supraventricular tachycardia and highly symptomatic, frequent ventricular ectopic beats.

One caveat: the success rates for ablation are generally lower for treatment of AFib, somewhere between 50 and 80 per cent,[6] so your heart specialist will need to know how long you have had AFib, the size of your heart's chambers and other factors when discussing whether this treatment may be right for you. Making lifestyle changes, particularly ones that can help reverse factors related to the metabolic syndrome (see page 59), may vastly increase the chances that your treatment will be successful. And in many cases improving your lifestyle is the only action needed to stop AFib episodes.

Case study: Robert

Over the years I've had many patients describe a clear association not just between large meals and atrial fibrillation, but between certain foods and changes in their heartbeat. The most unusual case I've encountered was Robert, who was in his mid-forties and whose AFib was triggered every time he got a takeaway Thai – not Japanese, or Italian, or any other type of cuisine.

Was it the monosodium glutamate (MSG)? An intolerance to lemongrass or some other ingredient specific to Thai cuisine? I don't know.

What I do know is that he reliably had AFib episodes when he ate Thai food for about two years, before developing regular AFib with less obvious triggers and heavier symptoms. At this point we decided that it made sense to do an ablation to cure his arrhythmia. He has not had any AFib since the procedure and now enjoys Thai food again.

It just goes to show how much we still have to learn about cardiac-rhythm disorders and their triggers.

Pacemakers: A pacemaker is an implantable device that generates and transmits an electrical impulse to a chamber of your heart. This causes the chamber to contract, leading to a heartbeat. These are small devices that consist of a battery, a computer circuit and one or more electrical wires called pacing electrodes that attach directly to the heart's muscle. They are usually implanted inside the body just below the left collarbone.

Pacemakers are typically implanted in people with low heart rates (bradycardia) who are experiencing dizziness, shortness of breath (dyspnoea) or fainting (syncope). It's important to rule out other possible causes of a slow heart rate that might be reversed without a pacemaker, such as low thyroid function, being cold and being on beta-blockers or calcium channel blockers (CCBs). Often treating the other condition, or stopping the drugs, will allow the heart rate to normalize and a complete resolution of symptoms. Low heart rates can also be caused by conduction tissue disease, which is typically seen in ageing hearts, or by damage to the muscle from a heart attack or muscle weakness (cardiomyopathy).

However, heart rates below 60 beats per minute are not reason enough to insert a pacemaker. It's very normal for fit, healthy adults to have heart rates dropping below this, especially during sleep. So long as you don't have dizziness associated with a low heart rate, this is usually considered to be normal.

Implantable cardioverter defibrillators (ICDs): You may recall seeing defibrillators installed in various spots around your town, especially in airports, schools and sports arenas. They are usually housed in boxes with the International

Liaison Committee on Resuscitation (ILCOR) defibrillator label – a green heart with an electric 'shock' symbol. If someone loses consciousness as a result of a very rapid heart rhythm (cardiac arrest), the electrode pads of a defibrillator can be placed on the chest and used to deliver a shock to the heart, restoring it to a normal rhythm. An ICD is essentially one of these devices packaged into a much smaller box and inserted inside your body, typically under your left collarbone. Your doctor may recommend an ICD if you have had a prior cardiac arrest or if your risk of a cardiac arrest in the future is deemed to be high.

ICDs are usually implanted in a specialist cardiac catheter laboratory. For a **transvenous defibrillator**, an incision is made under the collarbone, and the defibrillator – about the size of a stopwatch – is implanted. Electrode leads connected to the defibrillator are then threaded through a vein to the heart. If needed, electrodes may also be threaded to the left ventricle via a vein called the coronary sinus, to ensure that the pacemaker delivers an electrical impulse that keeps the ventricles beating in sync. With a **subcutaneous defibrillator**, the electrode leads are inserted underneath the skin rather than being threaded through a vein.

Regardless of what treatment you and your doctor choose for your arrhythmia, there are a number of things you can do to reduce the impact of your irregular heartbeat on your heart's health – especially understanding your triggers, keeping risk factors under control and treating obstructive sleep apnoea, if you have it. You can also be a true partner with your doctor by becoming more aware of your irregular heartbeats, whether through getting to know your typical pulse or by investing in a device that will record your heartbeats, if you can afford this.

Of course not all palpitations are associated with a rhythm disorder. They can sometimes be a precursor to a fainting spell – a condition related to the heart and blood pressure, which we look at in Chapter 6.

6. Fainting

Imagine a family gathering centred around a big feast – whether a Christmas or Thanksgiving lunch of roast turkey plus all the trimmings and roast potatoes; or a Korean harvest feast of braised-beef short ribs and sweet rice cakes, washed down with rice liquor; or a Persian new-year picnic of pilaf with fried fish and stuffed grape leaves. Food and drink have been abundant and everybody's rest-and-digest response is taking over, settling them into a contented late-afternoon doze. Then Gran says she's not feeling well, stands up, becomes light-headed and faints.

When she comes to, she's disoriented and complaining of palpitations. Some people think she may have had a fit or a heart attack. Others worry that she may have broken a bone in her fall. An ambulance is called and she is taken to hospital.

A few hours later, after a battery of tests, the doctor explains to a crowd of concerned relatives that their matriarch has post-prandial hypotension and has experienced syncope (pronounced 'sin-cope-pee'). What's that?

In this chapter we will learn how disorders of the heart and circulation can cause loss of consciousness and blackouts. This can be frightening, but once you understand why you are fainting and when you are prone to do so, you will have the power to protect yourself from injury.

What's the difference between loss of consciousness, blackout and syncope?

Loss of consciousness occurs when the area of the brain that maintains consciousness is impaired.

Head trauma, such as a hard fall or accident, can cause you to lose consciousness for a prolonged period. A cardiac arrest or stroke can interrupt the supply of oxygen to parts of the brain long enough to shut down the brain's consciousness centres. Severe infections in the brain and drug or alcohol overdoses can do this too. In these cases, loss of consciousness can last for hours, days or weeks, with people regaining consciousness in a hospital intensive-care unit.

The term 'blackout' is used to describe a transient (short-duration) loss of consciousness. Blackouts usually occur suddenly, with a rapid recovery, often within minutes. They can be due to:

- **Epilepsy**: a disorder of the brain
- **Syncope**: a disorder of the circulation
- **Psychogenic pseudo-syncope**: a complex disorder of the psyche, where there is an appearance of transient loss of consciousness, despite normal blood flow to the brain and normal electrical brain function.

In the past, researchers have estimated that about one-quarter of people diagnosed with epilepsy do not have epilepsy, but instead experience syncope.[1] Less than 1 per cent of people globally have epilepsy, in contrast to 40 per cent of people (or more) who will experience vasovagal syncope at least once in their lifetime.[2]

Vasovagal syncope is the term for an episode of blacking out due to low blood pressure, low heart rate or a combination of both these factors. Cardiac syncope, a potentially life-threatening cause of blackout, usually caused by impaired blood flow to the brain from a heart-rhythm disorder (see Chapter 5), is much less common, so our focus in this chapter is on vasovagal syncope.

Blackouts checklist

If you're having blackouts, consult a doctor to uncover the cause. Before your appointment, think about your history of blackouts, as this information will help in making an accurate diagnosis and developing the right treatments for you. It may be helpful to have notes on the following:

- **How often do you black out?**
- **What triggers your blackouts?**
- **How long does it take for you to recover?**
- **What were you doing one minute, five minutes, thirty minutes and four hours before the blackout?**
- **What medications do you take regularly?**
- **How much water, caffeinated drinks and alcohol do you typically drink each day?**
- **Do you have warning signs prior to a blackout? These may include dizziness, sweatiness, looking pale (pallor), palpitations or nausea.**
- **Does anyone in your family have a history of loss of consciousness or of sudden death before the age of sixty?**

To determine which of the three distinct reasons for blackout is causing you to lose consciousness, your doctor will review your medical history with you, will examine you and have you take some tests. Your history is the single most important diagnostic test in distinguishing between vasovagal syncope, epilepsy and other conditions causing loss of consciousness.

Vasovagal syncope versus epilepsy

	Vasovagal syncope	Epilepsy
History		
Description of blackouts	Blackouts that occur with warning signs lasting for several seconds or minutes; blackouts that occur only in sitting or standing positions; long-standing childhood tendency to 'faint'; tendency to black out in warm weather, crowded places, after a large meal (postprandial), when dehydrated or when having blood taken	Seizures with or without loss of consciousness
Symptoms	Nausea, blurred vision, distant hearing, rapid palpitations, panting-like breathing, feeling warm and needing to get 'fresh cool air'	Temporary confusion, uncontrollable jerking movements of arms and legs, repeated body motions such as lip-smacking or blinking, staring 'blankly' into space without a point of visual focus, fear, anxiety, a feeling of déjà vu

Triggers	Standing for long periods (which increases pooling of blood in the legs), standing up rapidly from a squatting or lying position, large meals, alcohol consumption, heat exposure, extreme fear, stress, anxiety, pain, having blood taken	Lack of sleep, fatigue, alcohol consumption, missing medications, stress
Clinical observations (examination)		
Blood pressure	Low (< 100/70mmHg) or low–normal (100–120/70–85mmHg); readings may drop lower when standing	Often normal; diagnosis usually made by history
Diagnostic tests	Electrocardiogram (ECG), twenty-four-hour portable ECG Holter monitor or echocardiogram (echo), exercise stress test, tilt-table testing	MRI brain scan and electroencephalogram (EEG)

What's happening in syncope

The most common form of syncope, **vasovagal syncope**, is called this because it links the blood vessels (vaso-) with the vagus nerve (-vagal), the information superhighway of the parasympathetic nervous system connecting the brain to the heart, the gut and beyond – to the bladder, skin, sweat glands and pupils of the eyes. This form of syncope occurs when the autonomic nervous system temporarily malfunctions in response to a trigger. As a result, the heart usually beats more slowly, the blood vessels dilate and blood pools in the large blood vessels of the gut and the legs. This can lead to low blood pressure (hypotension) and a slow heartbeat (bradycardia). Typically, if the blood pressure drops below 60/40mmHg, you faint.

When your blood pressure drops like this, you will immediately feel unwell. You may have palpitations and feel light-headed, dizzy, sweaty, clammy, nauseated or sick, before passing out. It may be possible to stop yourself losing consciousness if you quickly sit or lie down keeping your feet elevated.

Blackouts and your blood pressure

If you have invested in a blood-pressure measuring device (see page 21), you can take a collection of readings to see if you have low blood pressure (hypotension) or a drop in blood pressure due to changes in posture (orthostatic stress).

1. Take three readings (spaced over five minutes), all while lying down.
2. Take a reading immediately on standing up.
3. Take five readings (five to ten minutes after standing) with your legs shoulder-width apart and your arms by your side and not moving.
4. Note how you feel: dizzy, light-headed, head rushing, sick, totally fine?

If your blood pressure drops while you're standing to a low level (systolic blood pressure under 100 mmHg) and you have other symptoms, then it's likely that you have a tendency to experience vasovagal syncope. Share your readings and notes with your doctor.

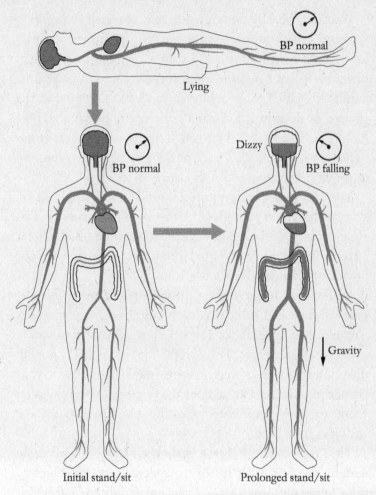

Lying

Dizzy

BP normal

BP normal

BP falling

Gravity

Initial stand/sit

Prolonged stand/sit

1. Gravity causes blood to pool into lower limbs
2. The heart is filled with less blood
3. Blood pressure drops, leading to dizziness, sweatiness, nausea and palpitations

What happens when you feel faint after prolonged standing/sitting

Blackouts may be the body's strategy to regain some blood pressure when your blood pressure is dropping to extremely low levels like this and you are sitting or standing in an upright position. When someone loses consciousness, muscle tone is relaxed, which often results in the body slumping to the ground or floor in a horizontal, or close to horizontal, position. The blood that has pooled in the legs due to gravity has a chance to return to the heart, pushing up blood pressure and improving circulation. Consciousness is restored.

You and your doctor can feel confident in a diagnosis of syncope based on your medical history, clinical exam and an ECG reading. If there is any doubt, you may be asked to wear a Holter monitor overnight to try to catch the rhythm of your heartbeat when you have a blackout.

You may be referred for a **tilt-table test**. During this test you will be asked to lie down on your back, face upwards (supine), on a tilting table. The table is then tilted, head up, to a seventy-degree angle. This forces blood to suddenly pool in the veins in your feet, which may provoke syncope due to your change in posture. Throughout the test your blood pressure and heart rate are monitored, allowing your doctor to observe any changes in them.

The graph overleaf shows vital observations for someone undergoing a tilt-table test for suspected syncope. Fluctuations in the person's systolic (top line) and diastolic (bottom line) blood pressure are shown. After five minutes of lying down, the table was tilted up (first vertical line). There was an initial rise in blood pressure, followed by the patient declaring symptoms of dizziness and nausea at 14 minutes (vertical symptom marker), with progressive worsening of symptoms

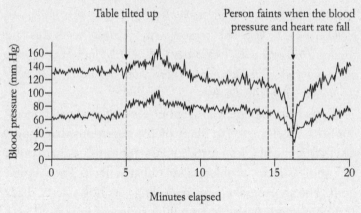

A tilt-table test of a person with vasovagal syncope

in the next two minutes until the blood pressure plummeted from 110/70 to 45/30, during which time the patient lost consciousness.

There is no such thing as a 'simple faint'

I have run the Imperial College London Syncope Diagnostic Unit, one of the largest syncope units in London, for more than ten years. I have reported more than 8,000 table-tilt tests and met even more patients.

This experience has demonstrated to me that, despite how common syncope is, it is almost always miscommunicated and misunderstood – by both patients and doctors. Whenever someone has an unexplained blackout with red flags, it should be treated as a medical emergency. When they faint regularly, they can seek treatment to reduce this – through lifestyle changes or, in some cases, drugs. But too many doctors tell their patients, *It's just a simple faint. Drink more water, stay cool and you'll be fine.* The person with syncope hears this and thinks, *The doctor doesn't know what I have! How can drinking more water help cure a life-threatening illness? How can staying cool cure a debilitating chronic condition?*

If you have experienced syncope recently, you will remember how it feels: *terrifying*. Many of the sensations that appear just before the blackout (prodromal symptoms) seem to point to a serious heart problem, like a heart attack. The palpitations. The shortness of breath. Feeling very hot, sweaty, dizzy and nauseated. A rising, spiralling sense of anxiety. These symptoms of stress are the product of your body's fight-or-flight reflex, kicked into gear because your blood pressure is falling too rapidly.

> ### Alert! Red-flag symptoms in syncope
> Certain symptoms that occur in syncope should be considered 'red flags' because they might be a sign of a heart-rhythm disorder or severe valve defect – cardiac syncope, a condition that may lead to prolonged loss of consciousness or sudden death.
>
> If you experience any of the following, seek urgent attention:
>
> - Syncope without warning
> - Syncope with injury
> - Syncope during exercise
> - Syncope preceded by abrupt rapid palpitations.

There is *no* such thing as a 'simple faint' – that's the campaign slogan of the Syncope Trust and Reflex Anoxic Seizures (STARS) charity. With so many people experiencing syncope over the course of a lifetime, we all need to learn more about fainting and how to prevent it. For this purpose I set up the website stopfainting.com, and I encourage you to visit it if you're interested in learning more about how you can stop fainting.

Preventing vasovagal syncope

If you are otherwise fit and healthy, without any other medical conditions, you can manage vasovagal syncope very effectively using a simple set of strategies.

- **Stay hydrated**: Drink plenty of fluids – aim for 2.5–3 litres (4½–5¼ pt) a day, enough that the colour of your urine remains pale.
- **Allow more salt in your diet**: This will help expand the volume of blood circulating in your body. When you take salt (sodium), you will also feel thirsty and drink more, and this will help to prevent dehydration. Be sure that you do not have high blood-pressure readings before you do this. It's worth noting that a majority of patients with vasovagal syncope have low–normal blood-pressure readings, typically between 100/60 and 110/70mmHg.
- **Avoid triggers**: Many common triggers are easy to avoid. Avoid standing for prolonged periods or standing up too

quickly, and lie down while having blood tests if you're prone to fainting during these tests.

- **Improve blood flow from your feet back to your heart:** Perform isometric exercises such as buttock-clenching or tensing of the front of the thighs and calves. This is akin to 'squeezing' blood pooling in your legs back up into your heart and brain. You might consider wearing compression stockings, which also encourage blood flow up from the legs back to the heart. Look for graded thigh-length or waist-height styles in grade 2 (25–35 mmHg).

- **Recognize your prodromal symptoms:** These are the symptoms that precede an episode. They may include feeling hot or getting dizzy. Act on them by sitting down, lying down or performing isometric exercises. If you feel you might pass out, sit down immediately – even if this is at a bus stop or in a supermarket queue. Doing so can avoid significant injury caused by falling.

- **Review your medications:** If you are taking hypertensive medications to lower blood pressure, these may need to be changed. Speak to your doctor.

If these simple measures fail to reduce fainting episodes, and your blood pressure remains low, then your doctor may choose to prescribe medications to augment your blood pressure. These may be drugs such as a vasopressor called midodrine, which works by tightening blood vessels, or the steroid drug fludrocortisone, which encourages your kidneys to absorb more salt. Both boost blood pressure and can minimize how often you have vasovagal syncope episodes.

The brain's power over the body

One of the most difficult to diagnose – and hard to manage – syncope conditions is **psychogenic pseudo-syncope**. This is different from syncope because there is the appearance of loss of consciousness rather than true loss of consciousness. To add to the confusion, there are numerous terms used to describe and diagnose it, including conversion disorder, non-epileptic attack disorder and functional syncope.

In psychogenic pseudo-syncope, a person has normal blood pressure, normal heart rate and normal electrical brain patterns. Yet despite this, there is an apparent loss of consciousness. Sometimes the blackout is accompanied by unusual movements or motor or sensory-function impairment.

It's not entirely clear why this occurs. Some people with psychogenic pseudo-syncope also have anxiety or depressive symptoms. There may be a traumatic event in the person's past that has made them more prone to having their emotional stress manifest in physical symptoms. But sometimes there are no obvious factors like this. How emotions can have such a powerful physical impact on the body remains an incredibly difficult concept to grasp and communicate.

The best diagnostic tool is usually medical history. If you are having frequent attacks, up to several times a day, it's far more likely that you are having psychogenic pseudo-syncope, since episodes of vasovagal syncope occur far less frequently. A tilt-table test that provokes symptoms, despite no significant change in your heart rate or blood pressure, can confirm your diagnosis.

Case study: Julia

Julia, a highly performing eighteen-year-old, walked into my office to discuss treatment for her symptoms of syncope. She had been fainting infrequently since childhood, typically during hot weather, especially if she was dehydrated – a clear case of vasovagal syncope. Her condition had become worse over the past year, after she had moved from home to start university and joined a rowing club. When she told me that her blackouts were now occurring only during term time, and several times a day, I put my pen down. It was time to stop scribbling notes and engage in an open and trusting manner, to allow Julia to express the full breadth of her story. This wasn't vasovagal syncope, but something else.

I encouraged her to tell me about how her expectations for uni were lining up with her experience. She shared that she was anxious about the challenges she was facing, both academically and as an athlete. She had been on her rowing team at secondary school, dedicating most of her time to training and competing, and had been a top performer. Now she feared she would not be good enough to participate in any races – some of the other club members were training to qualify for the Olympics. And she felt as though she was falling behind in her studies. The blackouts were making things worse. She thought she'd had her syncope under control.

We talked about how her brain was activating a 'circuit breaker', causing her to have symptoms that felt like her vasovagal syncope to her, but in reality were caused by entirely different mechanisms. This helped her to significantly reduce her psychogenic pseudo-syncope events within three months.

Living with syncope

Syncope is perhaps the most common cardiovascular problem, but it is eminently treatable.

Help your doctor make an accurate and correct diagnosis. When you see your doctor, take your filled-out blackout checklist. Ask your family and friends to tell you how you are when you have a blackout, so that you can share this information with your doctor. Consider purchasing a blood-pressure monitor (see page 21) so that you can record your blood pressure, along with your heart rate and other symptoms, while both sitting and standing. Most importantly, learn the red-flag symptoms (see page 104) and seek urgent attention if you have them.

Care for your body and yourself. Identify your triggers and avoid them, keeping in mind that stress can be an important trigger, no matter what kind of syncope you are having.

Remember that it's better to be embarrassed and conscious than to be injured and unconscious. This means that you need to take early evasive action when you feel the warning symptoms of a blackout – sitting or lying down immediately, no matter where you are. Make your safety your top priority.

Acknowledge your diagnosis and set yourself realistic expectations for recovery. Whether it's vasovagal syncope or psychogenic pseudo-syncope, acknowledging your diagnosis will be crucial in improving your symptoms. There may be some ups and downs on your journey to recovery, but you will get there. You can imagine a future without frequent fainting spells, and maintaining a sense of positivity about your prospects will help you successfully manage your condition over the long term.

7. Eating for a Healthy Heart

In the previous chapters we've seen how different conditions affect the heart and circulatory system. Along the way I've mentioned how making changes in your diet can significantly reduce the chances that a heart problem will become serious, and in some cases will actually stabilize or reduce an existing heart problem. While some of these changes relate to a specific condition – for example, cutting caffeine out of your diet, if you find it typically sets off palpitations – there are many ways in which you can change your diet to make your heart healthier more generally, giving it the fuel it needs to keep it ticking for longer.

Developing a 'heart-healthy' diet has long been one of the holy grails of medicine. Unfortunately, until quite recently the scientific community and government guidance have not always given people the best advice. It's time to change that and give you a better menu for supporting your heart's health.

Forget the food pyramid

Back in the 1940s an American doctor called Ancel Keys was worried about the number of his fellow countrymen who were succumbing to heart attacks. So he decided to look at the health and habits of men aged forty to fifty-nine across seven different countries – the US, Finland, Greece, Italy, Japan, the Netherlands and Yugoslavia (today Croatia and Serbia) – to work out what put some men's hearts at greater risk. The findings of the study convinced Keys that the diet of people in southern Europe was more protective to men's hearts than the diet eaten in northern Europe. And thus the so-called 'Mediterranean diet' – a moderate-fat, fresh-fish-heavy diet – was created.

It's worth noting that the Mediterranean diet in its purest form does appear to protect the heart. This is when the fats consumed are things like extra-virgin olive oil and olives, and pasta and breads are eaten in small amounts and made the old-fashioned way, from whole grains.[1] Of course diet is only one part of the jigsaw – other factors such as getting regular exercise, exposure to sunlight and good sleep, as well as having a strong sense of community, are now known to contribute to longevity. However, when the findings of the seven-country study were published in full,[2] the recommendations became distilled into a simple diagram: the food pyramid. You may remember these old pyramids, which often featured an overflowing bread basket at the base. It didn't help that many people incorrectly associated the Mediterranean diet with big bowls of spaghetti and sauces mopped up with loaves of bread. A craze for carbohydrate-based diets was born.

Fat, at the pinnacle of the pyramid, was squarely positioned as the villain, and many countries developed programmes to encourage people to start eating low-fat versions of foods to improve their health. Carbohydrates replaced fat in most people's diet, especially after it was alleged that eating foods high in saturated fats put you at higher risk of heart problems; carbs seemed to have the stamp of approval from health experts after all. The simplicity of the pyramid was so alluring that for many years the American Heart Association allowed food manufacturers to put 'heart-healthy' labels on boxed cereals that contained extremely high, unhealthy levels of sugar – often equivalent to a candy bar's – simply because the products were low in fat.

The advice to eat a low-fat diet has not improved people's health, however. People are getting fatter and sicker, and the number getting heart disease has continued to rise. In the early 1980s, when the UK's first low-fat guidelines were introduced, about 6 per cent of the population had a body-mass index (BMI) of 25 or more, classifying them as being overweight or obese. This figure has ballooned tenfold in the space of just over a generation, so that today, 63 per cent of UK adults are either overweight or obese – which means it's now more 'normal' to be overweight or obese than to be a healthy body weight. The World Health Organization has classed the rising incidence of obesity worldwide as an 'epidemic'. The chief executive of the NHS has called it 'the new smoking'.

Being overweight puts more strain on the heart, of course. But it's not just carrying weight that is impacting upon the heart. That fat building up on the belly (central adiposity) is associated with having more fat in the liver and pancreas, which is a root cause of insulin resistance and Type 2 diabetes. In other words, fat is a sign of something else happening in the body that puts the heart at risk.

Not all calories are created equal

Newer research has shown that in fact it's carbohydrates that we need to limit in order to lose weight and improve heart health.

This may seem counterintuitive if you are imagining plaques of lipids (fats) sticking to the walls of your arteries and 'furring' or 'clogging' them up. However, a calorie of protein or fat appears to have less inflammatory impact on your body than a calorie of carbs.

Why would that be? The building block of all carbohydrates is the sugar molecule **glucose**, which is the body's basic energy package for cells. When you eat carbohydrates such as bread, rice, potatoes, pasta and breakfast cereal, your gut breaks down these carbs into packets of glucose. This is quickly absorbed from your gut into your blood, so that when you eat carbs, the level of glucose in your blood increases rapidly – within thirty to sixty minutes of eating.

Your body doesn't like to have a large amount of sugar in the blood. So whenever the pancreas – a gland nestled between your stomach and your spine – detects a sugar rush, it produces the hormone **insulin**, which sends out a signal to your body's cells to absorb the excess glucose. This helps return your blood-sugar levels to normal. If many of your cells do not need an immediate energy boost – and they often don't, while you're in rest-and-digest mode – the body stores this energy for later use. Some of this glut of glucose is converted into glycogen and stored in your liver and muscles. The rest is converted into triglycerides and stored in your fat. So the more excess carbohydrates you eat, the more weight you gain. Food that is low in glucose but high in protein or fat does not increase your blood-sugar levels in this way.

With this in mind, let's consider a typical 'healthy' Western breakfast of a slice of dry brown toast, a bowl of bran flakes with milk and a glass of apple juice. The carbohydrate load of this meal will quickly be broken down by your gut into its glucose building blocks. In fact this carb-heavy breakfast will be broken down into the equivalent of sixteen teaspoons of sugar. Most of this excess glucose will end up as fat.

Teaspoons of sugar in a breakfast[3]

Food	Serving size	Teaspoons of sugar
One slice of brown bread	30g (1 oz)	3
Bowl of bran flakes	30g (1 oz)	4
Milk for the bran flakes	125ml (5 fl. oz)	1
Glass of apple juice	200ml (8 fl. oz)	8
Total		16

Worse, this breakfast sets you up for a day of storing fat, because the spike in insulin produced by your pancreas will eventually reduce your blood-glucose levels to a point where, a couple of hours after eating, your body starts looking for energy again. However, what you ate earlier is no longer easily accessible to fuel your cells; it's stored in your liver, muscles and fat. So you crave a snack. You might end up doing this all day long, putting your body through a roller-coaster ride of carbohydrate consumption and blood-glucose surges, followed by a surge of insulin to drive down blood sugar by locking glucose in your liver, muscles and fat.

Because of the anti-fat guidelines put out over the past several decades, many adults grew up eating this way, experiencing a series of sugar rushes during the day. Children's bodies are better able to use this sugar, because they are growing and their cells need energy continuously throughout the day. However, this conditions the brain to seek out sugar rushes too frequently, which appears to damage the heart in small ways.[4] And if we grow up getting used to being 'treated' (or treating ourselves) to a carb- or sugar-laden food like confectionary, chocolate or cakes, it can be very hard to break the association between sugar and comfort. But it's a habit that we need to break, for our heart's health – and a habit we should try to avoid bestowing on our kids.

The insulin effect

It gets worse. When you run on high-carbohydrate foods and don't take regular exercise to mop up the excess glucose, your body will produce extra insulin. High insulin levels actually prevent the body from breaking down fat into energy. So the more insulin your body produces on a regular basis, the more fat you store, the less fat you burn and the more weight you gain.

In addition, the body does not like being continually bombarded by insulin, either. Eventually, as a way to protect itself from this, many parts of the body, such as the liver, stop listening to the signal of insulin, becoming **insulin-resistant**. At first the pancreas tries to overcome insulin resistance by producing a lot more insulin, but eventually it gets to a point where it cannot produce enough. When this happens, glucose is no longer efficiently removed from the blood and your blood-glucose levels begin to run high. This is called **hyperglycaemia**. If hyperglycaemia persists over time, you will develop Type 2 diabetes.

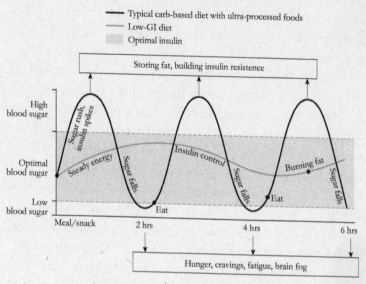

How a diet high in carbohydrates leads to
a roller-coaster of blood-sugar and insulin levels

The risk of developing Type 2 diabetes increases from the age of forty. Sadly, however, doctors are routinely seeing more and more people in their early twenties with this condition. It is also more common in some ethnic groups, including among people of African, Caribbean, South Asian or Middle Eastern heritage.

You may have diabetes without noticing any major symptoms. Sometimes the most obvious symptoms are needing to urinate more frequently, feeling thirsty, wounds healing more slowly and fatigue. Some people experience serious symptoms such as blurred vision and poor circulation before their diabetes is diagnosed. Untreated diabetes can lead to kidney (renal) failure, blindness and permanent nerve and circulation problems in the feet, which in some cases must be treated with amputation of the limb.

Having diabetes significantly increases the chances of experiencing a heart attack or heart failure. Long-term studies like the San Antonio Heart Study and the Women's Heart Study, which have followed groups of people over many years, suggest that the association between diabetes and heart failure may be due to increased inflammation. When the body has to regularly convert glucose into glycogen for storage in the liver or muscles, or into triglycerides for storage in fat, it can cause chronic low-grade inflammation in these tissues.[5] This seems to have a cascading effect, with inflammation occurring in other organs, including the heart and blood vessels.[6] Worryingly, you don't have to reach the levels of insulin resistance in diabetes to develop low-grade inflammation at levels associated with cardiovascular diseases; it is also seen in people with insulin overproduction without diabetes (pre-diabetes).

There are other ways in which developing Type 2 diabetes can affect your heart's health. People with diabetes tend to have not just more glucose, but also more triglycerides circulating in their blood. They have higher blood pressure and less good (HDL) cholesterol as well.

In most cases, Type 2 diabetes can be managed well – and even reversed – by changing your diet to be lower in carbohydrates and sugars and by increasing your physical activity, so that your muscles use up all the glucose in your blood straight away, before it gets stored. Exercise also lowers insulin resistance.

Low-glucose eating

To reduce the amount of glucose circulating in your blood, you don't need to cut out carbs completely from your diet. Carbohydrates are an important part of a balanced diet. Instead, you want to eat carbohydrates that break down into a lower amount of glucose.

The effect that foods have on your blood-sugar levels is captured in the glycaemic index (GI). Foods with a high GI cause your blood glucose to rise more rapidly, which provokes your pancreas to release more insulin. Pure glucose has a GI index value of 100. Anything with a GI value of 50 or higher is considered to be a high-glucose food. There are many GI index tables available online that offer average GI values. These are helpful for identifying the worst culprits, even though the GI value of a food can differ from person to person.

Some high-GI foods may not be surprising, although just how much sugar they pack may be shocking. Orange juice from concentrate has a GI value of 57, not much less than a can of cola, which comes in at 63. An orange is healthier at 40, but a grapefruit offers a much lower sugar spike with a GI value of 25. Beans and nuts, which are made up of carbohydrates as well as proteins and fats, all tend to fall under 50. Pizza has a very unhealthy GI of 80, and some types of potato rival pure glucose for GI value! Even some 'healthy' snacks, such as rice crackers, rye crisps, popcorn, watermelon and raisins, are considered high GI.

You want to aim to build your diet around foods with lower GI values, such as vegetables, fish, eggs, beans and nuts, a small amount of meat and some fruits, such as apples, peaches, pears and berries.

Breaking fast later

Every cell in your body contains its own built-in clock. Over a twenty-four-hour period, these internal clocks tell your body's cells what time of day it is generally. This is important because each cell is adapted to carry out certain functions at specific times of day. This includes eating.

Professor Satchidananda Panda of the Salk Institute in California pioneered the concept of eating according to your body's natural biological (circadian) clock, after discovering that the body is best able to respond to incoming food during a particular window of time lasting eight to twelve hours in every twenty-four. For the other consecutive twelve to sixteen hours, the body prefers to be in a non-eating (fasting) state.

In recent years a number of experts have urged people to adopt a programme of time-restricted eating, popularly known as **intermittent fasting**, based on Professor Panda's idea of circadian eating. Some advise skipping or significantly reducing meals on two days each week, with good health benefits. However, the evidence suggests that it is not necessary to go for a long period of time without eating, or to eat very restricted calories on certain days of the week, to get the health benefits of intermittent fasting. In fact you can tap into the metabolic advantages of intermittent fasting simply by breaking your overnight fast later in the day – that is, taking your 'break fast' later.

A review of evidence published in the *New England Journal of Medicine* found that by ensuring at least twelve hours between the last calories consumed at night and the first calories consumed in the morning, people were able to switch their body into burning energy stored in their fat as fuel, reducing their craving for glucose-rich foods.[7] Because the body is getting its energy from fat, the pancreas does not kick into gear to produce insulin. And during the fasting window, when there is no incoming food, there are no spikes in blood glucose, so insulin levels stay low, reducing inflammation in the blood vessels. It may seem paradoxical, but since I started to skip breakfast in 2019 I've felt a consistently high level of energy throughout the morning and far less craving for a snack before lunch. So, for your heart health, *when* you eat may be as important as *what* you eat.

Ketogenic diets aim to shift your body into a state where it regularly gets energy from the triglycerides stored in your fat – instead of from sugars that you have recently consumed – through a process called **ketosis**. When your body breaks down triglycerides in your fat, they are turned into ketone bodies – a more efficient fuel, compared to glucose, and in fact a source of energy preferred by the brain. So in addition to extending the 'break fast', proponents of ketogenic diets suggest substituting carbohydrates with very rich fats (for instance, coconut oil), on the premise that these will help your body run more on ketones than on glucose. However, the regime can be very hard to maintain long-term, requiring exacting diaries and measurements of the content of every piece of food consumed. Some of the suggestions for doing this are also culturally unfamiliar – like putting a pat of butter or half a teaspoon of coconut oil in your coffee, rather than a splash of milk – and 'keto-friendly' food products can be ultra-processed as well as expensive. Lastly, because carbohydrates are so drastically reduced, ketogenic diets are low in fibre, which could result in health problems.

For this reason, it is encouraging to see the very strong evidence for a more 'user-friendly', low-sugar and low-processed foods programme that has been developed by Dr Saira Hameed and her colleagues at Imperial College London. Called the **Imperial Satiety Protocol** (I-SatPro), it involves skipping breakfast and building your diet around low-GI foods – fish, eggs, beans and other legumes, nuts and seeds, healthy fats with cardiovascular benefits, full-fat dairy, some meat, non-starchy vegetables and certain fruits.[8] The programme focuses on educating people about the impact on the body of eating high-sugar foods, supporting them to break the roller-coaster of sugar spikes, insulin spikes and eventual insulin resistance, with all of the health problems that these bring.

In I-SatPro, participants aim for sixteen hours of fasting – so if you have your last food and drink at 8 p.m., you aim to eat and drink no earlier than noon the next day. Water, coffee and tea are allowed during the fasting window. (Although black coffee or tea is best, the I-SatPro programme does allow for a small splash of milk.) While this requires a big shift in how you structure your daily meals, it's easier to adopt in a shared household – especially if you have children – than some of the more involved ketogenic diets. And of course your kids can still have breakfast to fuel their day while you chat with them.

The people participating in the I-SatPro study have typically been overweight or obese and were referred to the university's weight clinic for help with complex weight and metabolic issues. Many have tried numerous diets and exercise programmes over the years, with no success. They've often said that, on previous plans, they found it hard to keep track of the rules – how many calories they could eat each day, or what percentage of their calories they could get from this or that food group. There is no calorie-counting in I-SatPro; instead, the focus is on restricting the hours when you eat and on reducing or avoiding high-GI carbohydrates like bread, rice, potatoes, pasta and breakfast cereal. The programme uses coaching methods to hand the power of making these changes to the individual: you are *choosing* not to eat certain foods because they cause a spike in your blood-sugar levels.

I-SatPro participants who stayed with the programme for one year lost 14 per cent of their body weight on average, which is similar to the outcome when having invasive gastric-band surgery, where a band or other device is fitted around the stomach to make people feel full sooner. In addition, blood glucose and triglyceride levels came down, good (HDL) cholesterol levels went up and blood pressure fell. Importantly, participants reported significant improvements in their well-being and mood. Taking control of your diet feels good.

But won't eating fat increase cholesterol?

Eating more fat does not necessarily produce more body fat, and not all fats have an unfavourable ratio of good (HDL) cholesterol to bad (LDL) cholesterol. In fact, eating healthy fats like extra-virgin olive oil, butter and full-fat Greek yoghurt is healthier than substituting equivalents like margarine spreads, which are made up of unhealthy artificial fats; or low-fat yoghurt, which may be bulked up with hidden starches and sugars.

Some fats should be avoided. Trans-fatty acids, also known as **trans fats**, are a type of unsaturated fat that occurs naturally in meat and dairy from cows, goats and sheep. In animal products, the amount of trans fat is quite low – around 2–9 per cent of all of the fat you consume – and this is fine when eating meat in portions no larger than the size of a deck of cards a few times a week. However, there are also synthetic (artificial) trans fats. These trans fats are added to vegetable fats so that they remain solid at room temperature – think of margarine or spreadable butter substitutes.

Synthetic trans fats have often been used by food manufacturers in ultra-processed foods because these fats are cheap and have a longer shelf life. Store-bought crisps, crackers, biscuits, pastries and cakes have typically contained them. Many fast-food restaurants depended on trans fats to keep their outlets supplied and churning out deep-fried food. Excessive sugars and trans fats are the true villains in the global epidemic of obesity and cardiovascular diseases. Further, studies have shown that synthetic trans fats ramp up your LDL cholesterol while having no impact on your HDL cholesterol levels. Without the balancing effect of HDL cholesterol, you are more likely to experience furring of your arteries and heart damage.

Dr Hameed gives her patients some easy rules about fat to remember. First, use fat in a regular and common-sense way that makes your food tasty and filling (satiating). In contrast to many keto approaches, this means one teaspoon of butter (not three) to make an omelette. Second, use fats that are good for you. If your great-grandmother ate it regularly, then the fat is likely to be naturally occurring (from plants or animals) and okay to eat.

Your great-grandmother's fats versus synthetic fats

Adapted from the Imperial Satiety Protocol's guide to fats.

Heart-healthy fats – your great-grandmother's fats	Unhealthy fats – because they use highly processed vegetable oils or synthetic trans-fatty acids
Butter and ghee	Margarine
Extra-virgin olive oil Coconut oil	Highly processed vegetable oils, such as corn oil and sunflower oil
Lard (animal-meat fat)	Vegetable shortening
Nuts, nut butters (a handful or teaspoon a day) and seeds like flaxseed (linseed)	Processed fried foods (chips, deep-fried fast food, doughnuts) Store-bought processed and ultra-processed snacks (crisps, crackers, biscuits, pastries and cakes)
Full-fat dairy, such as milk, yoghurt and cheese (about 100g / 3½ oz or 100ml / 3½ fl. oz a day)	Products labelled low-fat, diet or light/lite

You may now be wondering why the effect of sugar did not show up in the seven-country study of heart disease in men conducted by Ancel Keys. It may have! One of the food groups most strongly associated with increased death from heart disease in the study comprised pastries – a lovely combination of fats, sugars and carbohydrates. At the time of the study, people's diets were also lower in highly refined carbohydrates, such as white breads, crisps and crackers.[9]

Should you 'go vegan'?

More than a decade ago former US president Bill Clinton adopted a mostly vegan diet to help control his coronary heart disease. He has credited his diet, based partly on a programme developed by Dr Caldwell B. Esselstyn,[10] with helping him lose nearly 13.5kg (30 lb) and recover from bypass surgery.[11] His story has inspired many people to wonder if the best way to protect their health is to go vegan too. I have had several patients in my clinic ask about this option.

Adopting a vegan diet is not for everyone, particularly people sharing a household with devoted meat eaters or dairy lovers. (President Clinton is 'mostly' vegan, because he does eat fish once in a while.) You also need to be mindful of ultra-processed substitution foods and the potential for vitamin deficiencies. Be sure you get enough vitamin B_{12}, which plays a central role in nervous-system function. Also watch your iron levels to prevent anaemia.

Evidence suggests that you don't need to make such an extreme change in eating patterns to improve your heart's health. In one study, vegans who maintained a twelve- to sixteen-hour overnight fast had reduced rates of death due to heart problems – but the reduction was about the same as for semi-vegetarians who fasted overnight and ate non-fish animal meat once a week, rather than giving it up altogether. Both of these groups had lower heart-related deaths than fasting non-vegetarians, so if you are a big beef, pork or poultry eater, it's definitely worth reducing how much of these meats you eat. If you do eat meat, eat it in a way that fits with I-SatPro – some meat, lots of fibre (at least 30g / 1 oz per day) and, most importantly, avoid ultra-processed foods containing industrially manufactured ingredients that you don't understand.

Change when you feel full

You may recall from earlier that Japan was one of the countries in Ancel Keys's study. Although much of the attention focused on the benefits of the southern European diet compared to the northern European diet, the Japanese men in his study also saw lower rates of heart disease – in fact, they had the lowest rates of anyone participating. As Japanese eating habits became more Americanized, starting in the 1960s, the rate of heart disease in Japan went up. This suggested to researchers that there was something about the traditional Japanese diet that protects the heart even better than the Mediterranean diet.

The traditional Japanese approach to eating is exemplified in the practices of the people of Okinawa, an island off the coast of Japan that is known as one of the 'blue zones' of the world – a place where people live longer on average than elsewhere and enjoy excellent cardiovascular and metabolic health.[12] The Okinawans believe you'll be healthier if you build a habit of being satisfied with less food. This is captured in *Hara hachi bu*, the concept whereby you stop eating when you are 80 per cent full.

Many of us are used to eating until our stomach feels 100 per cent full. This means we are taking in more calories (and usually more carbohydrates) than our body needs, *especially* since the parasympathetic nervous system will soon settle us into rest-and-digest mode to help push food through our digestive system so that essential nutrients can be fully absorbed by the body. As you will remember, when we go into rest-and-digest mode, our heart rate and breathing slow down, conserving energy, which means that we are rarely eating to satisfy an immediate energy demand. In fact researchers have shown that when we start to feel hungry, it is almost always based on our habitual eating times, not out of an immediate need for energy. This is why breaking the habit of a morning breakfast can stick over the long term, when you make a commitment to it.

As you eat, the digestive system produces a number of hormones that signal to the brain what and how much you are eating. One of those hormones is insulin. But there are other hormones too, and some help to signal to the brain when you've eaten enough. However, there is a delay between when these hormones are released and when the brain receives and interprets the 'fullness' (satiated) signal. For example, two hormones, glucagon-like peptide 1 (GLP-1) and cholecystokinin (CCK), slow down the movement of food in the gut to increase digestion, and this makes us feel full, but not immediately – it can take ten to twenty minutes. These hormones' effect can also be somewhat drowned out by feelings of pleasure from eating tasty food or sharing a meal with loved ones, or habits of eating, such as finishing everything on your plate.

Like the Okinawans, you can learn to be more aware of the feeling of satiety, by eating more slowly and giving more attention to how the gut is slowing down and filling up, rather than the other signals encouraging you to continue eating. Practically, this means first learning how much food at each meal is just enough to make you feel fullness in your stomach, then decreasing your portion size by 20 per cent. You can also improve the sensitivity of the nerve cells that signal the feeling of fullness by burning more calories through exercise.[13]

A diet personalized for you

In this chapter we have seen the health benefits of seemingly divergent approaches to diet, from the low-GI, time-restricted I-SatPro programme, to going vegan. While each approach has benefits, you will need to find the plan that best suits the way your body works and your own individual genetic make-up. In the past, people have done this through trial and error, but it is now becoming possible to tailor dietary recommendations to your unique physiology and genetics, using technology that was previously only used in research studies, but is increasingly available to the public.

Broadly speaking, there are three emerging approaches to personalized nutrition: using your genetics, your gut bacteria or your personal GI index to develop a diet suited to your body.

1. **The relationship between your genes, your weight and your response to certain foods**: Although you can change your weight by watching what and when you eat,

genetics play a significant role. Indeed, your weight is as inherited through your genes as your height is. This might seem implausible, but consider that between 1875 and 1975 the average height of a British man rose by 11cm (5 in).[14] That was due to improved nutrition.

There is no one gene that controls your weight. Instead, certain genes each have a small, cumulative effect, with some genes influencing how you respond to certain foods. The most widely studied of these genes is one called *FTO*. People with a certain variant of the *FTO* gene tend to weigh more, and this is because their bodies prefer to run on high-sugar, energy-dense foods.[15]

You can now get your 'weight genes', including *FTO*, analysed by a DNA sequencing company. You might find it helpful to learn more about your genetic make-up and how it influences your response to certain foods. For example, if you find you have the variant of *FTO* that makes your body gravitate towards sugary junk food, this self-knowledge might help you rule out diets that are unlikely to work for you, no matter how much willpower you exert. A time-restricted diet might be a more effective option for you.

2. **Your gut bacteria's role in digesting different types of food**: Our digestive system is made up of millions upon millions of cells – and about half of them aren't even human cells, they're bacteria. The bacteria living in our gut (gut microbiome) play a role in digestion, helping to break down the food we consume. Everything you eat, the bacteria living in your gut also eat.

Over the last two decades there has been increasing research into how the gut microbiome influence many areas of people's health, from body weight, appetite and blood glucose levels, to inflammation, immune-system function, mood and behaviour. Early studies have started to look at how the specific bacteria in your gut determine how your body responds to carbo-hydrates, proteins and fats.[16] Several companies now offer analysis of the types of bacteria living in your gut, which can be identified from a stool sample, and then provide dietary advice based on this. My view is that this emerging science is an area to watch, but at this stage it's not yet sufficiently developed.

3. **Your individual blood glucose response to eating certain foods.** Glycaemic-index tables online can give you a broad sense of which foods will lead to more (high-GI) or less (low-GI) glucose ending up in your blood after you eat them. However, for any given food, individuals experience widely variable blood-glucose responses. So an orange could cause a large blood-glucose increase in you, but a minimal one in me.

By wearing a continuous real-time blood-glucose monitor such as Abbott Lab's FreeStyle Libre, you can learn how particular foods affect your body. After four to six weeks of records, you'll be able to see patterns – for example, you might discover that having a snack of a plum causes a spike in your blood glucose whereas an apple doesn't, or that chickpeas cause a moderate bump in your blood glucose while lentils cause hardly any rise at all. In this way you can construct a bespoke low-GI diet, enabling you to eat foods that you enjoy while keeping your blood sugar and insulin under control.

Case study: Suraj

Suraj, a sixty-five-year-old accountant, came to see me in my clinic. His angina attacks had previously been treated by using stents to open up the coronary arteries, and he was taking a statin for high cholesterol. He had poorly controlled Type 2 diabetes and, despite taking insulin injections, his blood sugar was running high almost all the time. He was overweight, with a BMI of 28, and so low in energy that he needed to take a daily afternoon nap, even when he was at work.

He told me that he was keen to make intensive lifestyle changes to get his health back on track. In particular he understood that his excess weight was putting a strain on his heart and that inflammation from his uncontrolled diabetes was worsening his coronary artery disease.

Suraj chose to follow the I-SatPro programme: low sugar, no processed foods and moderate fat. In addition, by purchasing a monitor that continuously measured his blood-glucose levels, he could see the real-time effect on his blood sugar of the food he was eating. His diet changes stabilized his blood-glucose levels, and within two weeks he was able to stop taking insulin injections. The blood-glucose monitoring also enabled him to personalize and fine-tune the I-SatPro advice. For example, he found that cherries caused a large increase in his blood glucose, but strawberries did not; his blood glucose remained stable when he ate kidney beans, but almost doubled in response to lentils.

After just four months Suraj had lost 13 per cent of his body weight and his BMI had fallen to 24 – in the healthy range. His blood tests showed that he no longer had diabetes and his cholesterol profile was normal. And his energy levels had increased dramatically. He was now cycling and walking every day, completely free from angina pain.

Five tips for heart-healthy eating

One of the three pillars of keeping your heart healthy is eating in ways that prevent inflammation in your blood vessels, support a healthy body weight and maintain cardiovascular health. This involves learning the importance of what, when and how you eat and upending common myths about which foods are bad for your heart.

1. **Choose to eat fewer carbohydrates and sugars:** Adopting a low-GI diet may be enough to stabilize your blood-sugar levels, reduce insulin resistance, help you lose weight and improve your heart's health. If this is not enough, I-SatPro may be right for you. Wearing a continuous, real-time blood-glucose monitoring device can help you identify your personal GI index and develop a diet of foods that you enjoy and that lead to lower increases in your blood-glucose levels.

2. **Consider time-restricted eating:** Aim to have your meals within a twelve-hour maximum window each day: for example, first food at 8 a.m. and no food after 8 p.m. Gradually reduce this eating window to eleven, then ten, then nine, then eight hours, if you are able to. This intermittent fasting will allow your body to spend more of its time in a low-glucose, low-insulin state, with benefits including weight loss as well as less inflammation. It can be a particularly powerful tool for people with a genetic predisposition to craving sugary foods.

3. **Don't be afraid of fat – but stick to natural fats, avoiding synthetic trans fats:** Avoid low-fat versions of foods, which often contain hidden carbohydrates or other ingredients that will spike your blood-sugar levels. Get protein from nuts, seeds, soy or fish, all of which are rich in healthy fats. This combination of protein and fat protects the heart. Aim to keep portion sizes of protein to about the size of a deck of cards.

4. **Clean out your fridge and kitchen cupboards:** Avoid all processed and prepared foods containing ingredients that you may not be able to assess. If there are any ingredients on the label that you do not understand, throw the food in the bin (and do not buy it, going forward). Skip most condiments if you eat out – although mayonnaise is often okay.

5. **Reset your satiety level to 80 per cent:** We tend to eat more than we need because meals are a social habit – a time to enjoy the pleasure of food and drink, as well as

the company of family and friends. Draw your attention to what your gut is telling you and stop eating sooner. The conversation over your meal can continue after you've put your utensils down.

8. Exercising for a Stronger Heart

Getting regular exercise reduces blood pressure, bad cholesterol levels and blood-sugar (glucose) levels. More than that, it lowers the risk of cardiovascular disease by 40 per cent *more* than we'd expect just from those reductions.[1] If we had a medicine that over-performed like that in making your heart healthier, you probably wouldn't hesitate to take it, even if it caused a few muscle aches. Well, exercise is that drug.

Depending on the current health of your heart and other health conditions, you may need to consult your doctor or heart specialist about the best ways for you to become more physically active. Many hospitals and charities offer exercise programmes specifically tailored to people with heart conditions. Exercise is an essential component in cardiac rehabilitation after heart attack and heart surgery. If you've had one of these, you will almost always be enrolled in a structured exercise programme under the care of your doctor and therapists.

In this chapter we'll focus on why exercise improves your heart's health outside cardiac rehabilitation, including the approaches to exercise that provide optimal cardio benefit.

Why exercise helps your heart

After exercise, the body does not simply return to its pre-exercise state. Instead a cascade of physiological changes happen as you recover from heightened physical activity, with some of these changes continuing for several hours after you do your last jumping jack for the day.

For example, your blood vessels remain dilated for a long time after exercise, lowering your blood pressure. Blood pressure goes down for a number of reasons. Parts of the aorta – the main tube leading out of the right ventricle to the circulatory system – are peppered with specialized cells called baroreceptors, which get stretched when blood pressure increases, as they do when the heart is pumping more quickly during a workout. When baroreceptors are really stretched, they send electrical signals (impulses) to inhibit the fight-or-flight reflex of the sympathetic nervous system and enhance the parasympathetic nervous system, which increases vagus-nerve activity. This relaxes the heart's pacemaker and blood vessels, slowing the heart down and reducing blood pressure. Therefore although exercise does temporarily raise blood pressure, over the long run working out lowers your blood pressure throughout the day, including when you're at rest.

You may be wondering why these baroreceptors don't fix persistent high blood pressure for us. These cells are sensitive to *relative* changes in blood pressure, so if your blood pressure remains elevated due to blood-vessel damage or chronic stress, the baroreceptors read that as the new normal and do nothing.

Exercising may also have a protective effect in cardiovascular diseases, diabetes and the metabolic syndrome, through a reduction in inflammation. People who exercise regularly and intensely appear to have lower levels of several substances that rise with inflammation (biomarkers), such as C-reactive protein and interleukin-6.[2] This may explain why exercise has such a huge positive effect on the health of people's hearts.

All of these reasons may help to explain the large body of evidence to support prescribing 'exercise as medicine', including for high blood pressure (hypertension), high cholesterol (hyperlipidaemia), heart attack, stroke, metabolic syndrome and Type 2 diabetes. For example, brisk walking for at least 150 minutes a week, alongside a reduced-calorie diet, lessens the risk of developing diabetes by about 60 per cent – nearly double the effectiveness of taking the anti-diabetes drug metformin.[3] Increasing physical activity by ten minutes a day appears to increase good (HDL) cholesterol levels by 1.4mg/dL (0.036mmol/L), reducing heart health risk by 2–3 per cent.[4]

So it's time to get moving.

Exercise tips for everybody

Not everyone has access to a gym or personal trainer. If you do, and you enjoy exercising in this way and manage to make it to the gym to do a workout at least three times a week, then stick with this – and well done! This is keeping your heart healthy.

For the rest of us, exercise can often feel like a chore or a burden, even if we remember how great we feel when we exercise regularly or remind ourselves how important it is for keeping us healthy. It's just one more call on our time in a stressful life. And often it's the call on our time that gets pushed to the side while we attend to something else that feels, and sometimes is, more important – preparing a healthy meal,

spending time with children or ageing parents, sleeping, seeing an important client or finishing a project on time at work.

I struggle with this myself. After a ten-hour day of seeing
patients on the ward or in my clinic, the last thing I want to do
is head to the gym or go for an hour-long run. I want to head
home and enjoy some time with my wife and kids.

This is why I believe it is so important to make exercise
accessible to everybody – and by that I mean *everyone* and
every *body*, regardless of their home and work life, age, physical capabilities or current weight. Very often people who
have not exercised regularly for a long time, those who are
older and those who are overweight or obese, who may find
exercise much harder because of their weight, say it is just
too physically difficult to do the programmes they see in the
media or that their doctor recommends to them. They sometimes get discouraged on hearing that they have to maintain
an elevated heartbeat for thirty to forty-five minutes in order
for their exercise to 'count' towards their weekly recommen-
dation. This is just too difficult. There are three pieces of
good news here, according to research by Dr Harvey Simon
of the Massachusetts General Hospital and Harvard Medical School:[5]

1. Even getting moderate exercise, including brisk walking,
   for fifteen minutes a day helps – extending people's lives
   on average by three years.
2. You don't have to do your exercise in one go.
3. Once you build up enough stamina to do high-intensity
   exercise, you can spend less time doing exercise, with as
   much or more benefit to your health.

What's the difference between moderate exercise and high-intensity exercise?

Intensity	How it feels	Examples
Light	No extra effort or little effort, with your breathing unchanged – easy enough that you could sing a song while you are physically active.	Leisurely stroll
Light to moderate	Some effort, with your breathing rate increased. You can still have a conversation with another person with no problem, however.	Purposeful walk up to the shops
Moderate	Moderate effort, with your breathing rate going up more. You can still have a conversation with another person, but you're catching your breath to do so.	Brisk walk, like you're in a hurry, as well as exercises such as sit-ups, body squats or jumping jacks done at a comfortable pace
Moderate to high	A lot of effort that makes you a bit out of breath, so it's hard to speak in full sentences.	Fast walk, jog or a run, as well as exercises such as sit-ups, body squats or jumping jacks done in timed repetitions

Getting physical

Depending on how old you are, or how much you like browsing old videos on YouTube, you might remember the legendary 1980s pop hit 'Let's Get Physical' and Jane Fonda working up a sweat in dayglo leg-warmers. To support cardiovascular health, you *do* need to get physical – but you don't need to take up a sixty-minute aerobics routine. In fact you want a combination of physical activities: moving more, strength training and intensive aerobic exercise called high-intensity interval training (HIIT). There are options for all of these that can fit into even the busiest person's day.

Moving more

For many people today, a typical day is spent sitting for hours – in front of a screen, behind a reception desk or at the wheel of a car or truck. Easy to moderate physical activity helps to tone the heart muscle; and the more we move, the less our blood pools in our legs and feet.

One commonly suggested goal is to take at least 10,000 steps a day. This is about 8km (5 miles), which, at a typical twenty-minute pace per mile, requires spending about two hours moving. This might be easily achievable for you if you choose to walk to some places that you would usually get to by driving or taking public transport – but it's not necessary to walk that far! A recent study, tracking the health of 16,000 older women, found that walking about 4,500 steps a day (about three kilometres or two miles) nearly halved mortality rates, and after 7,500 steps a day the health benefits plateau.[6] There are many smartphone apps, like MapMyWalk (mapmywalk.com) and Strava (strava.com), that can help you keep track of how far you walk (or jog, run or cycle), or you can purchase a simple, cheap pedometer to lace up on your shoes.

Moving more can also be achieved with smaller commitments, even during a day spent mostly sitting. Set a time once every hour to move for at least five minutes. For example, stand up and walk at least 100 paces. If you do this once an hour in an eight-hour workday, you'll be 18 per cent of the way to 4,500 steps a day. Double it and you will be one-third of the way there.

Then do some stretches, repeating each one five times. You can get your upper body going with:

- Shoulder shrugs
- Neck stretches
- Sky reaches.

Next, to get the blood pumping out of your legs and feet, try:

- Leg pumps (this exercise is often advised for long-haul flights to help prevent blood clots forming in the deep veins of the legs)
- Foot circles
- Thigh stretches.

If you cannot get away from your seat, you can do these stretches to promote blood flow from a chair too.

During your moving break, take the opportunity to fill up a glass or bottle with water. Hydrating after physical activity is important, and getting more water also improves blood pressure.

Time it takes: about five minutes every hour, and it can be done alongside other activities.

Strength training

As we saw earlier, a combination of aerobic exercise and strength training has been shown to improve many heart problems, so adding some simple strength-training exercises to your weekly routine will reap benefits.

When you hear the words 'strength training' you might imagine having to make a hefty investment in dumb-bells or other equipment. But strength training does not require any equipment; it requires nothing more than your own body weight.

Aim to do strength-training exercises two to three times a week. Simple exercises include:

- Push-ups (press-ups)
- Body squats
- Forward lunges
- Planks.

There are many other types of strength-training exercises, such as sit-ups, split squats, hip raises, side lunges, mountain climbers, shoulder presses, glute bridges and rows. Pick ones that work for you.

You can find videos online showing you how to do strength-training exercises and providing tips on how to avoid straining muscles and tendons while you do them. Be careful not to overdo it. You do not want to injure yourself so that you are unable to do the exercises regularly.

Speed is not the point in a strength-training workout. Focus on how the major muscles of your legs, arms, chest and shoulders are carrying your weight, giving them time to take on more weight, rather than on how fast you finish the exercises.

Start by repeating each type of exercise ten times. When this begins to feel easy, repeat each exercise twenty times. When this starts to feel easy, consider adding extra weight by holding something while you do the exercises – It does not need to be dumb-bells or other specialist equipment. It can be a couple of 1-litre (1¾-pt) milk bottles with handles, washed out and filled with water, or a couple of heavy books. It's best to have about the same amount of weight in both hands to ensure that you are working the muscles on both sides of your body equally.

Remember to hydrate after you finish.

Time it takes: ten to thirty minutes, two to three days per week

High-intensity interval training

High-intensity interval training (HIIT) is a great way to fit aerobic exercise into a busy schedule. Most importantly, studies show that it's an ideal way to keep your heart healthy. HIIT improves insulin resistance, reduces inflammation and increases cardiorespiratory fitness, and doing ten minutes of HIIT has been shown to provide the same cardiovascular benefits as much longer traditional workouts – for example, forty-five minutes of moderate-intensity cycling.[7]

HIIT involves a short burst of high-intensity exercise followed by a rest interval followed by another short burst of exercise, repeated several times. For example, one of the more popular approaches that has been studied by researchers – the 4x4 workout – involves a four-minute burst of high-intensity exercise, followed by three minutes of rest, repeated four times. In a lab the intensity of exercise is measured against the maximum amount of oxygen your body can consume in a minute, and is usually set high – between 80 and 95 per cent. What this means is that you want to go all-out for those four minutes.

HIIT workouts can be done while running or cycling, but you can also fashion a highly effective workout at home by doing some of the same exercises you do in your strength training: for example, push-ups, body squats and lunges. A HIIT workout might also include:

- Jumping jacks (star jumps)
- Circular arm swings (non-jumping jacks)
- Burpees.

You do a set of exercises for one minute, rest for one to two minutes, then exercise again, until you have done four or five sets. Some trainers suggest doing one type of exercise as many times as you can for a minute, switching to a different exercise in each set: so one minute of push-ups, rest, one-minute of burpees, rest, one minute of side lunges, rest, one minute of body squats. Others suggest doing five repetitions of exercises in sequence until you reach the one-minute mark: five push-ups, five burpees, five side lunges, five body squats, five circular arm swings. Then rest and repeat. Some programmes stick to a 4x4 workout of four minutes of exercises followed by rest, repeated four times. This takes about twenty-eight minutes – still half as long as Jane Fonda's old aerobics routine.

There is no particular best HIIT exercise programme – you have to choose one that works for you. I personally enjoy the Nitric Oxide Dump (nitricoxidedump.com) developed by Dr Zach Bush, which consists of squats, arm raises, circular arm swings and shoulder presses in a super-compact four-minute workout. That's easy to fit into a busy diary, even in between surgeries.

Aim to do HIIT exercises two to three times a week. And once you learn how to do the exercises, steal any time you can – for example, while waiting for the kettle to boil or vegetables to steam, or during a natural break between work meetings. You can do one cycle of exercise and rest at a time, spreading out your four or ten repeat cycles across the day. Soon enough you may be getting a daily hit of HIIT, and wanting more, because of how it lifts your mood and improves your health!

Time it takes: four to twenty minutes.

The wider benefits

Getting exercise has far-reaching health benefits. It can help with losing weight and appears to have a protective benefit against inflammation and a number of diseases, including cancers, osteoporosis, arthritis, chronic obstructive pulmonary disease (COPD), Alzheimer's, Parkinson's, depression and anxiety disorders.

It is also a great chronic-stress reliever, including in people with heart problems such as hypertension. Some researchers think this may be because the short-term stress of exercise helps train the body's autonomic nervous system to work more efficiently when it responds to stress.[8] Studies have found that people who get regular exercise experience lower increases in blood pressure during stressful emotional events.[9] The release of the feel-good hormone endorphin, often called the 'runner's high', after aerobic exercise may help too. People who do regular exercise also have more regular sleep patterns, which can reduce the effect of stress.

No matter why exercise helps, getting physical more regularly is an important tool in reducing and managing stress in your life – the third major pillar of a healthy heart.

Five tips for getting cardio-fit

It can feel like an uphill struggle to start exercising, or exercising more, if you've settled into a routine where you spend most of your time being sedentary. But you can do it, by taking small steps to start with and building up over time. You'll soon see how good it feels to make time for exercise, and your heart will thank you for it.

1. **Set an alarm to remind you to move at least once per hour:** It's easy to lose track of time and spend the day seated. But you need to keep the blood from pooling in your legs and feet by moving – getting up to walk and stretching.

2. **Create a personalized programme with exercises you enjoy:** I've suggested some strength-training and high-intensity interval training (HIIT) options, but there are many others to try if these specific exercises aren't for you. Try to incorporate all three elements across every week: moving more, strength training and HIIT.

3. **Fit exercise into your day so that it becomes part of your life**: If you create a programme that requires working out for an hour after work every Monday, Wednesday and Friday, the odds are that something will come up that conflicts with your workout at least a couple of times each month, if not more frequently. You want to make exercise a habitual activity that's as easy and regular as brushing your teeth.

4. **Don't get discouraged**. It will take time to improve your physical fitness if it's been some time since you have exercised regularly. You may feel out of breath, or imagine that it's not helping, if you aren't losing weight. But losing weight isn't the primary goal (and it requires changes in diet too). Even small amounts of exercise improve heart health. So keep with it, if only for fifteen minutes a day.

5. **Pay attention to how you feel**. Make a note of how you feel after exercising – you may be astonished at how much it lifts your mood and makes it easier to deal with stressful situations. This is good for your heart, but also for your overall well-being, and it might be the encouragement you need to exercise more frequently!

9. Creating a Better Balance between Stress and Rest

Over the millennia of human evolution, the stress response has kept generation after generation of people alive. Surging heart and breathing rates, eye-pupil dilation and increased blood flow to the muscles prepared our ancestors to successfully fight predators, prey, rivals and other threats – or to flee the scene to safety, when necessary. And after our ancestors managed to slaughter some ferocious sabre-toothed tiger or massive woolly mammoth and bring it home for a feast, they would sleep for many hours, perhaps even days. Under the thrall of the parasympathetic nervous system, their bodies enjoyed long stretches of rest, relaxation and rejuvenation between sudden but temporary bursts of adrenaline and cortisol.

Fast-forward to modern life – a period for which our automatic stress responses are less ideally evolved. Most of us now feel under continuous threat from things that are not so easy to escape. If a snake appears near where you're sitting, you run away or kill it, but once you've removed the threat, your heart and breathing rate quickly settle back down to normal. Getting pinged from the moment you wake until late in the evening by emails from your boss, becoming anxious about making your mortgage payments or paying your monthly bills, worrying about how you'll be able to care for your children or ageing parents, thinking about your own health, especially in

a world reshaped by the first global pandemic in a century –
these are stressors that can't be dispatched by running away
or grabbing a rock. In other words, modern-day living has
replaced intermittent, short-lived bursts of healthy stressors
with ever-present chronic stress.

Chronic stress puts us in a constant state of sympathetic
nervous-system activation, which in turn prevents the parasympathetic nervous system from expressing itself as often or
as completely as our body wants or needs to ensure that our
cells and tissues are resting and rejuvenating adequately. Much
more time in fight-or-flight mode and much less time in rest-
and-digest mode may be why people over the past century
have been experiencing higher rates of premature heart disease, high blood pressure, palpitations, digestion troubles such
as irritable bowel syndrome, sleep disorders like insomnia and
mental-health conditions like anxiety and depression. But it
also appears that chronic stress changes which **cytokines** – the
molecules that regulate how our immune system responds to
threats – become more responsive (upregulated). Those that
provoke inflammation are upregulated during chronic stress,
while those that reduce inflammation are downregulated.

The effect of acute versus chronic stress

Type of stress	Immune-system response	Impact on the body
Acute stress (less than two hours)	↓ Pro-inflammatory cytokines ↑ Anti-inflammatory cytokines	↓ Inflammation

Chronic stress	↑ Pro-inflammatory cytokines ↓ Anti-inflammatory cytokines	↑ Inflammation ↑ Susceptibility to infections, diabetes, depression and anxiety, cardiovascular diseases including hypertension, atherosclerosis and atrial fibrillation

Thankfully, there are ways in which we can give our para-sympathetic nervous system a boost, quieting our sympathetic activation. But first let's consider two ways in which stress takes a direct toll on the heart – 'irritable' hearts and 'broken' hearts.

Irritable hearts and broken hearts

During the American Civil War of the 1860s, physician Jacob Mendez Da Costa grew alarmed by the ravages of wartime that he was seeing in soldiers. Men were coming to him in droves complaining of headaches, diarrhoea, palpitations, dizziness, shortness of breath, anxiety and chest pains. What most alarmed him was what they had *not* experienced: physical injury in combat. All appeared physically fit and healthy on examination, and some had not actually participated in military action. Da Costa suspected that all of these soldiers had 'a disorder of the sympathetic nervous system'. He called it **'irritable heart syndrome'**.[1]

Over the next 150 years, through the two World Wars and the engagements in Korea, Vietnam, Afghanistan and Iraq,

a proportion of soldiers would return to civilian life report-
ing similar symptoms after service. They were diagnosed with
a range of conditions, depending on the understanding of
medicine prevailing in the day: shell shock, soldier's heart, cardiac neurosis, neurocirculatory asthenia, effort syndrome and
post-traumatic stress disorder (PTSD). What is common to
these syndromes is that their debilitating symptoms appear
to get worse when the person is standing upright. They suffer
from **orthostatic stress**, or stress provoked by changing position. For this reason, people who have headaches, diarrhoea,
palpitations, dizziness, shortness of breath, anxiety or chest
pains, with a heart-rate increase of greater than thirty beats
per minute on standing, are today said to have **postural orthostatic tachycardia syndrome** (POTS).

POTS is not exclusively a consequence of being sent to
war. Symptoms can appear shortly after physical or emotional trauma or a severe infection (the condition is neither
purely psychological nor purely emotional), and have been
observed in a wide range of people. During 2020 I started
seeing patients in the Imperial College Tilt Lab who were
experiencing symptoms such as diarrhoea, reflux, temperature dysregulation, anxiety, fatigue, rapid breathing and high
heart rates, frequently made worse on standing – all people
who had recovered from COVID-19 and showed no resid-
ual problems in their heart or lungs.[2] My colleagues and I
believe their symptoms are probably explained by autonomic
dysfunction in the wake of their SARS-CoV-2 (coronavirus)
infection – part of a syndrome being called 'long COVID'.

There is another way in which stress exerts a remarkable power over the cardiovascular system – **broken-heart**

syndrome, also called takotsubo (stress) cardiomyopathy, a disorder first described in Japan in 1990.[3] Most people with broken-heart syndrome have sudden chest pain (angina), shortness of breath (dyspnoea), fatigue or nausea, and when they go through tests at hospital, they have the classic diagnostic indicators of heart attack, including an elevated ST segment on an electrocardiogram (ECG); elevated levels of troponin, indicating damage to their heart tissue; and brain natriuretic peptide (BNP), indicating that their heart's chambers are over-stretched. However, on further examination these patients do not exhibit the physiological disorders usually associated with heart-attack risk, such as narrowed or blocked arteries. In fact, in most patients their arteries are smooth and clear. A heart scan shows the left ventricle has ballooned up, resembling the shape of a traditional Japanese octopus pot called a *takotsubo*, which is how the disorder got its formal medical name. For some reason, their heart muscle has suddenly weakened and stopped pumping normally – and that reason is stress.

Researchers have discovered that injecting large amounts of adrenaline into rats induces the characteristic ballooning of the animals' heart chambers.[4] This suggests that high concentrations of stress hormones may be what triggers the acute impairment of the heart muscle.

The stress triggers of broken-heart syndrome can be physical or emotional. For example, cases have been reported after the death of a partner, big arguments, surprise parties, extreme fear, a significant medical diagnosis, job loss, divorce, domestic abuse, shock, physical assaults, car accidents, over-exertion, major surgery, sepsis, asthma attacks and infection with the virus that causes COVID-19.

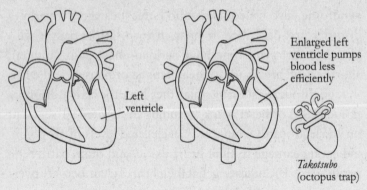

Enlarged left
ventricle pumps
blood less
efficiently

Left
ventricle

Takotsubo
(octopus trap)

Normal heart   Broken-heart syndrome

A normal left ventricle alongside an enlarged left ventricle
in broken-heart syndrome and a *takotsubo*, the octopus
trap that gave the syndrome its medical name

Women are much more likely to have an attack than men,
with 90 per cent of cases occurring in women, and it's more
common in women aged fifty or older and in those with a
history of head injury, epilepsy, anxiety or depression. Having one episode of broken-heart syndrome may indicate a
susceptibility to the disorder, as about 20 per cent of people
experience an attack more than once. Although the attack –
like a heart attack caused by a ruptured arterial plaque – can
cause death, in the vast majority of people (about 95 per cent)
it is temporary, with the heart returning to normal function in
a matter of days, weeks or months.[5]

Could stress-related heart syndromes be treated by short-
circuiting the nervous system's influence over the heart and
blood vessels? This is a subject of much research. Small

studies have been conducted to see if stimulating the vagus nerve – the complex of nerves that governs the parasympathetic nervous system and connects the brain with the heart and the gut – might help control a range of disorders, including epilepsy, anxiety, depression, headaches and pain, with mixed results.[6] Stephen Porges, an expert on vagal regulation, has investigated a far less invasive way to activate the parasympathetic nervous system: yoga.[7]

Porges and other scientists have been looking at how yoga and yoga-like activities can be used to regulate the nervous system through top-down and bottom-up processes.[8] **Top-down processes** involve the flow of signals from the brain to the body – the conscious or subconscious shift of the brain's attention and intention. These can be regulated by becoming more aware of your thoughts or emotions, and by actively guiding your attention and intention back to where you want it to be. **Bottom-up processes** involve the flow of signals from the body to the brain – the ways in which you can control your rate of breathing, posture and movement, which are cornerstones of yoga and yoga-like practices – to regulate your heartbeat and improve the balance between the two sides of the autonomic nervous system.

The autonomic nervous system's control over key body functions is essential to keeping us alive, but this does not mean that you can't exert some control over these automatic processes. And in my view, cultivating an ability to influence your autonomic nervous system is vital to improving your heart's health.

One way you can do this is through your breathing.

The ancient art of breathing

Most of the time you breathe in and out without much thought. You may notice your rate of breathing increasing, and may even feel short of breath, when you exert yourself, like when you do a set of reps in your high-intensity interval (HIIT) training. Your rate of breathing also increases if you're frightened or stressed. When you're resting and digesting, your breathing slows down.

It is now increasingly understood from a scientific perspective that our breathing regulates the balance between the body's fight-or-flight reflex and its rest-and-digest mode. Changing how you breathe sends bottom-up feedback to the autonomic nervous system, shifting it from fight-or-flight towards rest-and-digest. It's also easier to get into and maintain a state of emotional self-regulation and calm – what I call your 'heartset'. Finding this heartset through slow, mindful breathing sets off a cascade of other changes in your body, including the release of beneficial hormones that have restorative effects throughout the body.

This isn't an entirely new concept. In 1935 a French cardiologist called Thérèse Brosse headed off to India to study traditional meditative practices. In the palace at Mysore she met the guru Tirumalai Krishnamacharya, often called 'the father of modern yoga'. Krishnamacharya claimed that his breathing exercises had given him such control over his body that he could temporarily stop his heart beating. Brosse hooked the guru up to an ECG and watched in amazement as his pulse slowed until the recording needles seemed to still completely for several seconds.[9]

Although you may not perform as well as the guru of Mysore did, you *can* regulate your heartbeat through breathing and biofeedback – a technique that involves using touch, visual or auditory feedback to modulate the autonomic nervous system, in order to gain control of bodily functions such as heart rate and blood pressure. This is one of the best stress-management tools available and it takes just three minutes.

Learn to regulate your pulse

1. Feel your pulse for thirty seconds, giving it your fullest concentration. This means no emails, no talking, no texting, no watching TV or YouTube. It may help your focus to close your eyes.
2. Carefully notice the regularity of your pulse. Don't bother to count your pulse rate. Pay attention instead to how you're able to change your pulse rate.
3. After thirty seconds, take a deep breath from your belly to fully expand your lungs. Then let all the air out, slowly.
4. Next, slow down your breathing rate. Breathe in slowly for five seconds, then breathe out for five seconds. If you cannot manage five seconds, try three seconds, gradually increasing the time you take on each breath.
5. Return your attention to the regularity of your pulse. Notice the subtle changes in your heart rate with each rise and fall of your breath.
6. Bonus step 1: Start to imagine the following: *I am self-regulating my body through my breathing, and I am allowing the power of these breaths to infuse my*

heart, body and mind with optimal health. It may be easier to hear these words, or words like them, in your mind or by speaking them aloud.

7. Bonus step 2: Your breathing won't just slow your pulse; it will also lower your blood pressure. You can see this if you have a home blood-pressure monitor. Take your blood-pressure reading once, then breathe at a steady pace for three minutes, then take another reading. Your monitor will show consistently lower readings after slowing down your pulse.

Regulating your breathing is a robust, but typically untapped physiological tool for improving health and well-being. It improves respiratory sinus arrhythmia – what, in plainer language, is called **heart-rate variability** (HRV). In people with coronary artery disease, hypertension, heart failure and other cardiovascular disease, training in breathing and biofeedback pulse-regulation techniques has been shown to reduce stress and improve health outcomes.[10]

In his bestselling book *Breath*, James Nestor says that the 'perfect' breath has a 5.5-second inhale followed by a 5.5-second exhale. Some researchers believe this breathing cadence is ideally calibrated to quieten, or downregulate, the fight-or-flight reflex and activate, or upregulate, the rest-and-digest mode, but there's not enough evidence to suggest that inhaling or exhaling for a bit less or more time has a different effect. So start by inhaling and exhaling for however long feels comfortable for you, slowing down your breathing to slow down your pulse and improve your HRV. I find inhaling for eight seconds and exhaling for eight seconds to be most enjoyable for me.

Being more mindful

When we experience stresses, our brain and body unleash a chain of automatic reactions, releasing stress hormones, increasing heart rate, increasing breathing rate, and so on. It's easy to get pulled into the rushing current of these bio-chemical and physiological changes, going along with them until you hit an area of rocky rapids – a health crisis caused by chronic stress. But we can train ourselves to turn off the 'autopilot' response of stress through mindfulness-based stress reduction.

The field of mindfulness was developed in the 1970s by Jon Kabat-Zinn, a professor at the University of Massachusetts Medical School. A long-time yoga and Buddhist-meditation practitioner, he recognized that these practices would be help-ful for his patients experiencing illness, pain and anxiety, as well as chronic stress more generally. During mindfulness meditations, you take time away from the demands of life and focus on paying attention to your breathing, the sensa-tions in your body, your movements and the immediate world around you.

You also pay attention to your thoughts and feelings – but mostly to notice that they are intruding on the present moment. This is because our minds are constantly running scenarios: reliving past events or imagining future ones. That's a useful and necessary skill for learning and planning, and indeed is a major driver of human society and civilization, because it allows us to consider the effects of our behaviour and identify ways to improve it going forward. However, it can be hard to turn off! And the mind is powerful: our body often responds to the mental versions of our past and future just as it responds to the present, by releasing stress hormones, increasing heart rate and everything else. So mindfulness involves becoming more aware of our thoughts and feelings, and spending more time in the here-and-now.

Most practitioners advise that it takes several weeks of regular half-hour practice to rewire the brain from its regular habit of thinking about the past and future to paying attention to the present. However, you can start by practising being more mindful of a daily activity. Think about some short task that you normally do on autopilot, like brushing your teeth, having a shower, doing the washing up or eating a snack. Every day when you turn to this task, stop the autopilot and bring your full sensory attention to it. What do you see, hear, feel and taste? When you find your mind wandering into thoughts or feelings – what your boss said in an email, your excitement about an upcoming holiday, whatever it is – notice that, but then set it aside for another time. Bring your attention back to the present moment and what you see, hear, feel and taste. Really be present.

At first this might be challenging. You might start to reprimand yourself for your lack of presence. That's another way the mind gets distracted into the past, by judging ourselves for failures – even failures just a few moments previously. Set that judgement to the side too. It will take practice to let go of the past and future, and even the most experienced mindfulness practitioners don't let go of them entirely; they just get more efficient at noticing these thoughts and feelings intruding and setting them aside, so that they are less likely to have stress hormones build up.

Being in the present moment has significant benefits. People who have been taught to do transcendental meditation for fifteen minutes a day are about half as likely to die from heart attack and stroke, and they have lower stress levels and lower blood pressure.[11]

Keeping cool

There's an old idiom about the benefits of maintaining a sense of calm in moments of stress – keep a cool head in a hot situation. It sounds like a metaphor, but there might be something in applying it literally.

One of my favourite accounts of the benefits of yoga to physical health comes from Alexandra David-Néel, an explorer who lived to the age of 101 years. In her book *My Journey to Lhasa*, published in 1927, she shared almost unbelievable stories of how a meditative breathing technique called *tummo* had kept her body warm in the freezing temperatures of the high-altitude Tibetan plateau. A more modern take on this has come from Wim Hof, a Dutch man who holds several Guinness World Records for endurance feats, including the longest time immersed in ice – for more than one hour, forty-two minutes – and the fastest half-marathon run barefoot on ice and snow: in two hours, sixteen minutes. Although he has no formal training in meditation, Hof appears to have rediscovered something similar to the technique described by David-Néel almost a century ago.

Hof's method combines the use of cold to bolster changes in breathing and mindset. One exercise has you turn off the hot-water tap at the end of your shower for a shock of cold water – a practice that I've taken up and find invigorating, particularly when the cold water starts to feel warm against my skin. People with POTS often feel much worse in a warm environment, and some of my patients have reported feeling better with cooler showers and keeping the room temperature at home lower than their family members can tolerate.

Wim Hof also suggests practising holding your breath for as long as you can, three to four times in a row. When I do this, I can feel all my senses kicking into a state of extreme alert around the two-minute mark. Counting the seconds, 2:01, 2:02, 2:03, my brain, lungs and heart start to feel as though they are burning. I push on to 2:12, 2:13, 2:14 . . . and then I cannot hold my breath any longer. I take a sharp, deep inhale and quench my hunger for air. The results are almost instant: I feel relief more than anything, and my screaming senses calm down immediately, within the span of a single breath in and breath out.

Surely, you must be thinking, activating the sympathetic nervous system in this way is *creating* stress, and stress leads to inflammation – and that's not good. In my personal opinion, these exercises simulate the sort of sudden bursts of sympathetic nervous-system response that were regular features in the lives of our evolutionary ancestors, which may help to train the body to turn off stress quickly, rather than letting it hang around and become chronic. This is probably the closest most of us will ever get to the feeling of having a sabre-toothed tiger pounce on us – and without the actual threat of being eaten!

The shock from sudden cold or a prolonged breath hold can exacerbate heart irregularities. So if you have a pre-existing heart condition, do discuss the Wim Hof method with your doctor before embarking on it.

Getting a good night's sleep

When we sleep, our parasympathetic nervous system holds the reins. Studies have shown that having a consistent sleep cycle – between seven to nine hours a night, on a regular schedule – is essential to regulating the body's immune responses,[12] and sleep is good for your heart's health. Growth hormone – the hormone that promotes healing in the body – surges at night while we're sleeping. This hormone is key to restoring the lining of our blood vessels when they are damaged.

On the flipside, getting insufficient sleep leads to higher blood pressure,[13] and people who get fewer than six hours of sleep are two to three times more likely to have atherosclerosis.[14]

In addition, sleep deficiency seems to be associated with a higher risk of developing insulin resistance, the metabolic syndrome and diabetes. People with Type 2 diabetes are more likely to suffer from chronic sleep deprivation, getting fewer than six hours of sleep a night on a regular basis. It appears that when people get short sleep, their body is more likely to grab fuel stores from muscle than fat.[15] And in experiments, researchers have discovered that people deprived of sleep lose their hunger controls, eating on average 300 more calories the following day compared to what they crave after a good night's rest.[16]

Other feedback loops get set in motion when it comes to sleep and stress: stress can cause insomnia, and sleep deprivation causes stress;[17] and getting more exercise, which reduces stress, improves sleep.

It's not only important to budget time for sleep; it's also important to prepare your brain and body for bedtime. That means really turning off and tucking in. Mobile-phone use in the half-hour before you go to sleep, or even just keeping the phone near your bed, has been shown to disturb sleep and lead to poor sleep quality and a shorter sleep time.[18]

So commit yourself to a regular bedtime and wake-up time, and give yourself thirty minutes to a full hour to wind down at night. No screens, no phones, no planning for the next day. I find doing a mindfulness breathing exercise is a great way to ready myself for a good night's rest.

Building community and compassion

As human beings, we're not designed to be by ourselves. Our health and well-being depend on others. People with strong social supports are better able to manage stress[19] and have lower blood-pressure levels.[20] Those with a weak sense of attachment to close intimates and a lack of feeling of being part of their community (social integration) have higher rates of heart disease.[21]

Loneliness is a threatening state of being. Over time, it decreases our sense of mattering – meaning, mattering to others – and self-esteem, leading to the chronic stress and anxiety that can drive inflammation and associated diseases. This is why US Surgeon General Vivek Murthy has said that he considers loneliness to be an emerging health crisis. He has made it a mission to include information on local social groups and activities as part of public-health campaigns on how to improve the risk of illness and injury. He prescribes volunteering and service to others as an antidote to loneliness. These activities put us in touch with others and shift our focus from ourselves to someone else. They create the feeling that we are valuable and contributing to our world.

Feeling compassion makes us, and those around us, feel good, but it also has powerful effects on health and longevity. Julian Abel, a consultant in palliative care, argues that compassion is a more effective intervention for improving health outcomes than telling an individual to quit smoking or drinking, change their diet or get more exercise. He is part of the Compassionate Frome Project, a remarkable community initiative aimed at ending loneliness in the English town of Frome in Somerset, home to some 28,000 people. GP practices created a directory of local groups that bring people together – choirs, exercise groups, creative-writing workshops. They trained 'community connectors' to help guide residents to resources that would help them address problems, such as mounting debt or the need to find housing or simply socialize. In the wake of building these connections between 2013 and 2017, emergency hospital admissions have dropped by 30 per cent – at the same time that admissions in surrounding areas went up by 17 per cent. People in Frome report that their quality of life has also gone up.[22]

Interestingly, the benefits of connection and community may be related to a different form of stress response called 'tend and befriend' that has been studied by the psychologist

Shelley Taylor.[23] During psychological stress, the hormone **oxytocin** is released. This hormone is associated with the human impulse to seek the comfort of others, and to give comfort to loved ones and allies. Higher levels of oxytocin are seen in mothers immediately after labour and are believed to help mothers bond with their newborn child. Being able to turn to a support network of family and friends appears to reduce the effect of adrenaline and other fight-or-flight hormones, so that a response to a stressor might not be to fight or flee, but instead to tend and befriend. Further, research indicates that the release of oxytocin in the absence of family and friends leads to more and greater stress, creating a negative feedback loop. So in moments of stress it helps immensely to reach out to friends and family, either literally or figuratively.

Attending to your heart, from the heart

We all live busy lives filled with stressors and demands. Does anyone feel they have 'enough' time to do everything they want to do, every day? And everybody has a limited amount of energy to draw on in a day. I myself know this all too well.

In early 2020 I was speaking to my brother, who was sharing his journey into spirituality and suggesting things for me to read, and practices to do to bring a better balance into my life. At some point I stopped listening to him and my head filled up with all the demands on my time and energy. 'I don't have the time to do it,' I told him abruptly. 'You don't understand how many patients I see, how much research I do, how many emails I receive. I don't have enough time for my family.' I went on. The list of excuses I proffered was perfectly real and valid, but when I finished speaking, I had a moment of recognition: my narrative of excuses was no different from the stories my patients told me when I urged them to change their lifestyle to focus on their health and well-being. I knew making these lifestyle changes was an urgent matter for my patients with serious heart conditions. It's just as urgent for those who do not have, or don't yet know they have, heart disease.

This realization inspired me to put together a set of stress-management exercises that even the busiest person can make time for – and then I tested them in my own life, with the reasoning that I couldn't advise people to do something that I couldn't make time for myself. Here are three exercises to start every day – expressing heartfelt gratitude, focusing on your breathing and setting a healthy goal – plus a stress reset to do at intervals.

Express heartfelt gratitude

Instead of focusing on whether you have enough or not enough time, enough or not enough energy, choose to make time each day to bring your attention to things that really matter – that is, the things for which you are thankful. And be grateful for them. This is because gratitude is one of the strongest positive emotions, and research has shown that feeling gratitude improves happiness, health and well-being.[24] Raising this positive emotion first thing in the morning through a gratitude wake-up exercise can help to set your mood and frame of mind for the rest of your day, lowering your stress levels and increasing feelings of calm, connection and contentedness.

When the alarm goes off in the morning, many of us immediately reach for our phones to check in on what has happened while we were sleeping: the missed emails and messages, the overnight news, the change in the day's forecast. Or we start making an inventory in our heads of the things we must get done in the day ahead. Frequently this message-checking and job-list building sets off a spike in adrenaline – an immediate panic response, moments after we have roused from our restful slumber, pulling us away from the present blissful moment of waking up.

When you wake up, mentally push aside the phone and your to-do list and instead bring to mind your what-I-already-have list:

1. Lying in bed or sitting up, think about what you feel grateful for. This could be as simple as having had a good night's sleep, waking up next to a partner who loves and knows you intimately, enjoying your work or being able to walk in a nearby park or field.

2. Now think about who you feel grateful for. This could be your partner, caring parents, siblings or children, a wider network of family, friends, neighbours or colleagues, an understanding boss, friendly and attentive people working at the local supermarket or workplace. Spread your net of gratitude as close or as far as your mind likes.

3. Now let a feeling of deep gratitude for these things and people wash over you. Marvel at the wonder of your life, and feel joy in having these things to be thankful for.

Time it takes: three minutes.

Focused breathing

Now dedicate some time to breathe – just breathe – before you start your day. This doesn't need to be the exercise on learning to regulate your pulse on page 157 or any other specific meditative breathing exercise learned from yoga, mindfulness or other training. It can simply be a time when you let yourself breathe in and breathe out at a comfortable, slow rate, focusing your attention on nothing more than the regularity of your breath.

Whether you're simply breathing or paying attention to and slowing your pulse while you breathe, I suggest breathing for no less than three minutes. This will give you time to settle out of your thoughts of gratitude and into mindful attention to your breathing, activating your parasympathetic nervous system.

You can, of course, spend more time on breathing if your day allows – I typically devote ten minutes every morning to this part of my wake-up routine, breathing in for eight seconds and breathing out for eight seconds, again and again. When I was starting out I used a great biofeedback tool for Android and iPhone called Inner Balance from HeartMath (heartmath.com) to help guide my breathing over this span of time. The app allowed me to see my HRV change in real time in response to my thoughts, feelings and breathing pattern. When I noticed intrusive, stressful thoughts and feelings arise during my breathing, my heart rate became more jagged and unsettled; when I was able to express feelings of deep gratitude throughout the breathing exercise, then a stable, healthy HRV pattern arose and persisted, sometimes for several minutes after the exercise, coupled with a much longer-lasting sense of wellness. Seeing this has been a revelation, helping me to grow more personally aware of stress in my life and the benefits of both the gratitude exercise and time devoted to breathing.

My old, stressed-out self would have considered it a waste of time spending ten minutes each morning simply to breathe. But this has grown to be the most important part of my daily routine, setting me up for a fulfilling and productive day. (Visit drboonlim.co.uk/heart-healthy to see how breathing can directly create a healthy HRV pattern.)

Time it takes: three to ten minutes.

Set a healthy ambition

After feeling gratitude, focus on what you would really like to achieve on this day.

People who set goals feel greater motivation, self-esteem and confidence and they endow their actions with meaning, connecting what they do with a desired outcome, such as improving health.[25] They are more likely to succeed in reaching their outcome than those who do not regularly set goals for themselves. People who write down their goals appear to be more likely to achieve them; and telling someone you trust about your goals and then letting them know how you've done – feeling accountable to someone else – also increases the likelihood of success.[26]

I suggest choosing a single, deep-seated, empowering goal that puts you slightly outside your comfort zone – something like adding to your training routine a new HIIT exercise that pushes your physical fitness, or reaching out to someone you haven't spoken to in some time, to connect personally. Set your sights on something you can accomplish over the next twelve to sixteen hours – a goal that keeps you more in the present rather than thinking about plans for the future, and that binds you to doing whatever you can to meet your goal *today*.

1. Sitting up, think of one goal that you want to accomplish before you go to bed at the end of the day.
2. Check yourself. Is it something you can do in the next twelve hours? You want something you can accomplish.
3. Motivate yourself. Connect your goal to a higher purpose, such as improving your heart's health.
4. Commit yourself. Now write down your goal and, if you have someone you can share it with, tell them too. Use your written goal as a reminder not to let the demands of your day push it aside.
5. Check in. At midday do a goal check. Can you make time for your goal now, if you haven't already accomplished it? Then, about three hours before bedtime, check in again – and make time for your goal before the day ends.

Time it takes: one to two minutes to set the goal; how long it takes to achieve it depends on your goal!

Stress reset

You can also unwind stress during the day using a sixty-second 'stress reset'. This can be done any time – whenever you feel stress rising in you or have a free moment in your schedule.

1. At the start of a minute, inhale and exhale over ten seconds.
2. Continue this until your minute is over, keeping your attention centred on your breathing.

You'll be amazed at how different you feel after performing this exercise. It immediately dials down the stress reflex.

Time it takes: one minute, as many times each day as you like.

A better balance

Again and again when I talk with patients in my clinic, they have chronic stress in their life – usually a combination of personal, work and social stress that exists at a consistently high level, week in and week out. Yes, it's possible to treat some heart diseases with drugs or procedures, or to improve your health by eating better and exercising more, without tackling the things that send you into a state of anxiety or frustration. And in some cases what's making you anxious or frustrated won't be within your control. But you can take control of how long and how strongly you feel the effects of stress and what toll it takes on your body. Don't let one more day pass saying that tomorrow will be the day you get serious about changing your lifestyle to better reduce and manage stress.

Five top tips for creating a better balance

Establishing a better psychological and emotional balance in life is vital to physical health and well-being. Making the change now, starting with just three minutes of breathing, will improve your heart and your health, immediately.

1. **Create a daily routine**: Routines are powerful tools for improvement, as they enable you to create a habit out of stress reduction. You can set a routine including any number of intentions: for example, to do your wake-up gratitude, breathing and goal-setting exercises; to leave for a destination ten minutes earlier than you need, so that you can walk an extra block or stop on your way; to remove all mobile devices from the dining table during a family meal; to turn off your work devices at a set time in the day to enable you to focus on your family, your personal hobbies, your health and yourself; or to wind down one hour before bedtime – no exceptions.

2. **Slow your breath**: Spend time breathing slowly more often during the day. Breathe in this way when you wake up, when you notice you're getting stressed or emotional, when you're getting ready for bed and whenever you find you've got a free minute or two. You may also find longer breathing meditations, like the ones in yoga or mindfulness meditation, to be helpful.

3. **Observe more**: Spend time paying more attention to the present moment – the wind on your skin, the colour of the sky, the sense of sitting grounded in your chair, the emotions that rush over you when you think of a cherished loved one (or a deadline), the rate of your breathing and heartbeat. Mindfulness exercises are designed to help train your mind to focus more on the present versus the past and the future, reducing the impact of chronic stress. But it's also good for your

health (and lowers stress levels) to observe what you have to be grateful for – and to relish those positive feelings every day.

4. **Exercise more**: Being physically active is a great stress-reliever. It helps by putting the adrenaline released by the sympathetic nervous system to work for the purpose that nature intended – moving your limbs and getting your heart pumping, with a short burst of healthy physical activity. HIIT workouts are great for this, training your body to quickly shift out of fight-or-flight mode – something that also happens when you cap your workout with a shower in the Wim Hof way, with a shock of cold water.

5. **Get a good night's sleep**. There are so many ways in which sleep, stress and immune function are interrelated that it's essential to make seven to nine hours' sleep a night a goal for everybody.

10. Caring for Your Heart, Holistically

More than 90 per cent of cardiovascular disease is caused by how you live your life. Even among the 10 per cent of people with a high genetic susceptibility to particular illnesses, there is 50 per cent less risk of developing cardiovascular disease when they follow a lifestyle focused on maintaining a healthy body weight, eating a healthy diet, exercising regularly and reducing the impact of stress.

This is why I believe that shifting your mindset and heartset is the most important element in your health and well-being.

A positive mindset and heartset

Most improvements in health arise from putting *attention* and *intention* towards healthy lifestyle changes. And so I congratulate you – you're already paying greater attention to your heart's health by learning about how the heart works and what you can do to make it healthier. Now it's time to commit to having a firm intention to change your mindset – investing time, energy and other resources into ensuring that you take the knowledge you've gained and make it part of your everyday approach to living. Acknowledging the importance of emotions, and how these have a direct measurable influence on heart health, will help to improve your heartset – the heart-centred emotional state that defines how we respond to situations.

It's easy to fall into the trap of thinking that your time and energy are too squeezed to hold yourself to a promise to change the way you eat, exercise and manage stress. You might be thinking, *How can I stick to healthier food choices when I'm so busy that I can barely find twenty minutes to sort the shopping, let alone plan and prepare a balanced meal with fresh ingredients? Why is this diet going to help me lose weight, when I haven't succeeded in my previous three attempts? How can I ever find time to move and exercise more when I'm working twelve-hour shifts? And if I feel squeezed for time and stressed about eating better and exercising more, when am I going to practise breathing and mindfulness? My boss doesn't offer meditation breaks.*

Acknowledge these thoughts and see them for what they are: reasons not to change the way you're living and caring for yourself. Think about the people you love and who love you – your partner, children, parents, siblings, wider family and friends. Then think about all the things you'd still like to do in life: places you'd like to see, books you'd like to read or write, personal bests you'd like to achieve, promotions you'd like to earn, businesses you'd like to launch, events you'd like to witness or attend – including, perhaps, your first big personal project during retirement, a golden anniversary or the birth of a grandchild or great-grandchild. Really visualize them.

Now, with these motivations squarely in your mind's eye, tell yourself:

- *My health is one of the top priorities in my life.*
- *My heart is the top priority of my health.*
- *My heart's health is non-negotiable.*

The 'four Es' of holistic heart health

When I reflect on the journeys of my most successful patients – whether they are recovering from heart attack, over-coming POTS or reversing Type 2 diabetes – I've noticed that they share four characteristics. These aren't common physical or genetic types; instead, they are common ways in which they commit themselves to the lifestyle changes that will improve their health. I call these the 'four Es' of holistic heart health: education, expectation, empowerment and execution.

1. **Educate yourself**: My most successful patients learn about their illness and its causes, making and accepting the connections between what they do and how they feel. I've seen such good results from nourishing people's curi-osity that I now 'prescribe' learning to patients, in tandem with drugs or surgery. This might be reading a book on living a long, happy life, such as Héctor Garcia and Francesc Miralles's book *Ikigai: The Japanese Secret to a Long and Happy Life*, listening to Dr Rangan Chatterjee's *Feel Better, Live More* podcasts or watching a TED talk about the power of the placebo effect.

   Cultivate curiosity – a willingness to learn some-thing new every day – whether it's about your body's physical health or some other topic that will buoy your emotional and psychological well-being, such as the history of the community where you live, or how to play a musical instrument that you've always loved listening to. Approach making changes in your diet, exercise and stress management as an educational experience: a commitment to learn and develop not just new habits, but new skills.

Learning new things promotes feelings of wonder, joy and accomplishment and the sense of being fully present in the moment, without being distracted by the past or the future. Think of a time when you were so completely immersed in an activity that you lost track of time, unaware that hours rather than minutes had passed. Or recall the unbridled look of joy on a toddler's face when taking their first few successful steps and suddenly realizing that they are on their way to walking. That elevation in mood and mindfulness of the moment is something all of us can experience, no matter how old we are, our station in life or the condition of our bodies – and it's good for our heart.

2. **Expect a better future:** My most successful patients carry a realistic, optimistic expectation of recovering from their illness. This isn't unique to my clinical experience. A review of studies of people with cardiovascular disease found that those with a positive psychological outlook and a sense of optimism about the future were more likely to have good health outcomes.[1]

Martin Seligman, the founder of the field of positive psychology, argues that optimism isn't about putting a happy spin on your situation, but is instead about how you think about the causes of your situation. Do you think you're at fault (pessimist) or that you did what you could and might do better (optimist)?

Do you think you're stuck where you are (pessimist) or that things can change (optimist)? Being an optimist has significant benefits for your health. Optimists are more likely to learn about lifestyle risk factors for diseases[2] and then make lifestyle changes and seek support to help them change.[3] Optimism even seems to inoculate you, to some degree, from the inflammation commonly caused by stress.[4]

Happily, Seligman also believes that optimism can be learned, by stepping back from situations and looking at them through an optimist's eyes: *That wasn't my fault and I could do better. Normally things like this do turn out better; that was just a momentary setback.* Visualizing your 'best possible self' – what your life will be like in the future when you fulfil your ambitions – is incredibly powerful too.

So find something to aim for every day, and adopt an attitude of optimism towards achieving it. You will!

3. **Empower yourself**: My most successful patients choose to be an active and equal partner in developing and realizing the treatment of their illness. They see their lifestyle changes as being as important as – and often more important than – traditional medical interventions. Because they have learned about their condition and its causes, they want to share how they're improving their diet, exercise and stress management; and to be honest about where they're struggling, so that they can enlist my help. Together we can identify ambitions and develop a plan that fits their lives. And just talking through what they're experiencing is a stress-reliever.

Depending on your doctor's mindset, this might be a challenge. We doctors need to change our mindsets, too! If you attend my clinic presenting with hypertension, the simple solution would be to double-check your blood pressure and prescribe the latest evidenced-based medication. This takes all of three minutes: job done. However, what if you were struggling at work, having relationship difficulties, eating unhealthily, not exercising and getting only four hours of sleep at night, due to stress? If I didn't ask you about these triggers of hypertension, and you didn't volunteer the information, they would be missed. The prescribed medication might work for a while, but your unresolved triggers would continue to take their toll on your health, perhaps in other ways.

That's why engaging in an open, honest discussion with your doctor is so important, and why, in time-strained health services, you often will need to take the lead. Embrace an attitude that *you* are the person who must change your life, enlisting your doctor as your helper, where necessary. This will be empowering.

4. **Execute your plans**: My most successful patients do something meaningful every day. They are motivated to improve their health and well-being, but understand that they have to work to do so.

A big ambition such as improving your health and well-being can feel overwhelming to tackle. It can be more effective to break your plan down into what Arianna Huffington, the founder of *The Huffington Post*, calls 'microsteps' – steps that are 'too small to fail'.[5] The idea is based on research by the social psychologist Roy Baumeister of the University of Queensland, who discovered that making very small changes in self-control (for example, reminding yourself to sit up straight) increases willpower in other areas.[6] Repeat a change like this regularly and it becomes engrained behaviour – a habit.

Neuroscientist Daniel J. Levitin expounds that conscientiousness – a dedication to reliably performing at the best of your ability, whatever that ability may be – is the single most important personality trait in determining how well you age. So think about how you can push yourself to do more, and do it better each time that you set your mind to it.

Trying to regain fitness and health after a heart attack may involve small steps like taking a daily walk, breaking your fast a half-hour later each morning or getting an extra half-hour of sleep each night. As you chart out your meaningful microsteps, be sure to include ways to create connection with the people in your life – be they family, friends, colleagues or your wider community. Grow a beautiful garden, like the Okinawans do, that others can enjoy, or go out for a walk in nature, greeting passers-by with an infectious smile, no matter your mood.

Just writing a list of small, simple-to-execute changes in your daily routine can be the first microstep you take to improving your health. The next day pick a microstep from your list to be your second.

You control your heart health

My ideal world is one in which the public puts me 'out of business' as a cardiologist because they've adopted the sort of lifestyle choices that keep the human heart robust and healthy 90 per cent of the time. A world where people are curious, conscientious and empowered – and living a life full to the brim with gratitude and compassion for themselves and others.

I believe a focused mindset, regulated by a positive emotional 'heartset', has the potential to manifest unlimited abundance in health and well-being. So tap into that power. Take action, one step at a time, knowing and expecting that the changes you make can, and will, keep your heart healthy. The time to start making these changes is right now. Don't regret the past or fear the future. Embrace every moment and live life as if it were rigged in your favour, being ever optimistic. And know that you are in control of your heart health, your happiness and your well-being.

Top ten tips for a healthy heart

1. **Learn to check your pulse: Practise the sixty-second pulse check (see page 15) on yourself and others. This will help you sense when your heart is racing – an indicator of stress. If you have palpitations or very irregular rhythms, consider investing in a product like the KardiaMobile or Apple Watch, which record medical-grade ECGs (see Chapter 5) that you can share with your doctor to ensure early diagnosis and treatment.**

2. **Monitor and control your blood pressure: Buy an accurate upper-arm-cuff blood-pressure monitor (stridebp.org) and know your blood-pressure reading (see Chapter 2). Be sure to get high blood**

pressure (hypertension) treated urgently, since it may not cause any symptoms until you experience a serious cardiovascular event such as a heart attack or stroke. If you are fainting regularly, it's also worth seeing if your blood pressure is low and treating this (see Chapter 6).

3. Know your cholesterol and keep it at a healthy level: Do take up the opportunity to get your cholesterol checked as part of regular health screenings. If your cholesterol is elevated, educate yourself on the strategies to reduce cholesterol and your overall cardiovascular risk by making lifestyle changes (see Chapter 3).

4. Know your QRISK score: Your QRISK score (qrisk.org) will help you understand your risk factors for heart attack in an easy-to-digest format (see Chapter 4). As you fill it out, consider which lifestyle factors you have control over (such as stopping smoking) and focus on making changes in these areas.

5. Know your body-mass index (BMI) and aim to get it, and keep it, in the healthy range: Buy an accurate scale and use an online calculator to log your BMI (kg ÷ m²). Losing weight and lowering your BMI may take time, but resist the temptation to try extreme diets, which can be hard to sustain. Realize that you *can* make sustainable changes to what, when and how you eat, which will support weight loss and improve your cardiovascular health (see Chapter 7).

6. **Learn more about the impact of diet on your cardiovascular risk:** Eating high-sugar foods leads to fat storage, promotes inflammation and increases your diabetes risk. Cut out foods with a high glycaemic index (GI) value, and try skipping breakfast and eating only to 80 per cent fullness (see Chapter 7). These changes are often much easier to put into practice than you imagine, and the benefits may be seen within just a few weeks.

7. **Work some exercise into your daily routine:** Exercise can help condition your heart muscle, keep your arteries elastic and reduce stress. Stealing five to ten minutes at a time to perform high-intensity interval training (HIIT) – for example, doing a quick set of squats, push-ups and sit-ups while waiting for the kettle to boil – is a quick way to introduce a dose of exercise into your daily routine (see Chapter 8).

8. **Aim for seven to nine hours of sleep:** Appreciate that sleep is an investment in your health and well-being: it boosts immunity and productivity, sharpens the mind and promotes longevity (see Chapter 9). If you snore or are waking frequently during the night with a start, talk to your doctor about screening for obstructive sleep apnoea (OSA), which can lead to chronic heart problems (see Chapter 5).

9. **Breathe slower and deeper:** Deep-breathing stress-reduction exercises – breathing five

seconds in and five seconds out, for two to ten minutes – dials down the fight-or-flight reflex, helping to short-circuit stress before it becomes chronic. This will reduce your risk of high blood pressure (see Chapters 2 and 9).

10. Believe in your ability to manifest an improvement in heart health: With a positive mindset, you can start making microsteps, *right now*, to improve your heart health, your happiness and your well-being.

Notes

1. How Your Heart Works

1 William Harvey, *De Motu Cordis* (1628), in full: *Exercitatio Anatomica de Motu Cordis et Sanguinis in Animalibus*, trans. as *The Circulation of the Blood and Other Writings* by Kenneth J. Franklin, 3rd edn (London: J. M. Dent, 1968)
2 A. Popel (2017), 'Theory of oxygen transport to tissue', *Critical Reviews in Biomedical Engineering*, 17 (3), pp.257–321, www.ncbi.nlm.nih.gov/pmc/articles/PMC5445261
3 A. D. Waller (1887), 'A demonstration on man of electromotive changes accompanying the heart's beat', *Journal of Physiology*, 8 (5), pp.229–34, doi.org/10.1113/jphysiol.1887.sp000257
4 V. A. Cornelissen, J. Vanhaecke, A. E. Aubert and R. H. Fagard (2012), 'Heart rate variability after heart transplantation', *Journal of Cardiology*, 59 (2), pp.220–4, pubmed.ncbi.nlm.nih.gov/22266458

2. High Blood Pressure

1 B. M. Egan, S. E. Kjeldsen, G. Grassi et al. (2019), 'The global burden of hypertension exceeds 1.4 billion people: Should a systolic blood pressure target below 130 become

the universal standard?', *Journal of Hypertension*, 37 (6), pp.1148–53, pubmed.ncbi.nlm.nih.gov/30624370

2 GBD 2017 Risk Factor Collaborators (2018), 'Global, regional, and national comparative risk assessment of 84 behavioural, environmental and occupational, and metabolic risks or clusters of risks for 195 countries and territories, 1990–2017', *The Lancet*, 392 (10159), pp.1923–94, doi.org/10.1016/S0140-6736(18)32225-6

3 T. Unger, C. Barghi, F. Charchar et al. (2020), '2020 International Society of Hypertension: Global hypertension practice guidelines', *Hypertension*, 75 (6), pp.1334–57, www.ahajournals.org/doi/10.1161/HYPERTENSIONAHA.120.15026; K. Asayama, L. Thijs, Y. Li et al. (2014), 'Setting thresholds to varying blood pressure monitoring intervals differentially affects risk estimates associated with white-coat and masked hypertension in the population', *Hypertension*, 64 (5), pp.935–42, pubmed.ncbi.nlm.nih.gov/25135185

4 Unger, Barghi, Charchar et al. (2020), 'Global hypertension practice guidelines'

5 E. M. Sulaica, J. T. Wollen, J. Kotter and T. E. Macaulay (2020), 'A review of hypertension management in black male patients', *Mayo Clinic Proceedings*, 95 (9), pp.1955–63, doi.org/10.1016/j.mayocp.2020.01.014

6 A. Grillo, L. Salvi, P. Coruzzi et al. (2019), 'Sodium intake and hypertension', *Nutrients*, 11 (9), p.1970, www.ncbi.nlm.nih.gov/pmc/articles/PMC6770596

7 N. L. Benowitz and A. D. Burbank (2016), 'Cardiovascular toxicity of nicotine', *Trends in Cardiovascular Medicine*, 26 (6), pp.515–23, www.ncbi.nlm.nih.gov/pmc/articles/PMC4958544

8 A. MacDonald and H. R. Middlekauff (2019), 'Electronic cigarettes and cardiovascular health', *Vascular Health Risk Management*, 15, pp.159–74, www.ncbi.nlm.nih.gov/pmc/articles/PMC6592370

9 K. Husain, R. A. Ansari and L. Ferder (2014), 'Alcohol-induced hypertension', *World Journal of Cardiology*, (5), pp.245–52, www.ncbi.nlm.nih.gov/pmc/articles/PMC4038773

10 A. A. Thorp and M. P. Sclaich (2015), 'Relevance of sympathetic nervous system activation in obesity and metabolic syndrome', *Journal of Diabetes Research*, 2015, art.341583, www.ncbi.nlm.nih.gov/pmc/articles/PMC4430650; L. Landsberg (1986), 'Diet, obesity and hypertension', *Quarterly Journal of Medicine*, 61 (236), pp.1081–90, pubmed.ncbi.nlm.nih.gov/3310065

11 Anon. (2020), 'Social isolation during Covid-19 pandemic linked with high blood pressure', *Science News*, 19 November 2020, www.sciencedaily.com/releases/2020/11/201119083923.htm

12 J. H. Markovirz, K. A. Matthews, M. Whooley et al. (2004), 'Increases in job strain are associated with incident hypertension in the CARDIA Study', *Annals of Behavioral Medicine*, 28 (1), pp.4–9, pubmed.ncbi.nlm.nih.gov/15249254

13 T. W. Smith, B. N. Uchino, C. A. Berg et al. (2009), 'Conflict and collaboration in middle-aged and older couples', *Psychology and Aging*, 24 (2), pp.274–86, pubmed.ncbi.nlm.nih.gov/19485647

14 A. Steptoe, L. Brydon and S. Kunz-Ebrecht (2005), 'Changes in financial strain over three years, ambulatory blood pressure, and cortisol responses to awakening',

Psychosomatic Medicine, 67 (2), pp.281–7, pubmed.ncbi.nlm.
nih.gov/15784795

3. Bad Cholesterol

1 D. S. Wald, J. P. Bestwick, J. K. Morris et al. (2016), 'Child-
parent familial hypercholesterolemia screening in primary
care', *New England Journal of Medicine*, 375, pp.1628–37, www.
nejm.org/doi/full/10.1056/NEJMoa1602777

2 M. Tomaniak, Y. Katagiri, R. Modolo et al. (2020), 'Vulnerable plaques and patients', *European Heart Journal*, 41 (31),
pp.2997–3004, doi.org/10.1093/eurheartj/ehaa227

3 Ibid.

4 K. Moore, F. Sheedy and E. Fisher (2013), 'Macrophages in
atherosclerosis', *Nature Reviews Immunology*, 13 (10), pp.709–21,
www.ncbi.nlm.nih.gov/pmc/articles/PMC4357520

5 R. Y. Khamis, A. D. Hughes, M. Caga-Anan et al. (2016),
'High serum immunoglobulin G and M levels predict
freedom from adverse cardiovascular events in hypertension', *EBioMedicine*, 9, pp.372–80, pubmed.ncbi.nlm.nih.
gov/27333022

6 A. P. Kithcart and J. A. Beckman (2018), 'ACC/AHA versus ESC guidelines for diagnosis and management of
peripheral artery disease', *Journal of the American College of
Cardiology*, 72 (22), pp.2789–801, pubmed.ncbi.nlm.nih.
gov/30497565; F. Mach, C. Baigent, A. L. Cataano et al.
(2020), '2019 ESC/EAS guidelines for the management
of dyslipidaemias', *European Heart Journal*, 41 (1), pp.111–
88, doi.org/10.1093/eurheartj/ehz455

7 A. D. Gepner, M. E. Piper and H. M. Johnson et al. (2011), 'Effects of smoking and smoking cessation on lipids and lipoproteins', *American Heart Journal*, 161 (1), pp.145–51, www.ncbi.nlm.nih.gov/pmc/articles/PMC3110741

8 J. A. Finegold, C. H. Manisty, B. Goldacre et al. (2014), 'What proportion of symptomatic side effects in patients taking statins are genuinely caused by the drug?', *European Journal of Preventive Cardiology*, 21 (4), pp.464–74, doi. org/10.1177/2047487314525531

9 R. R. S. Packard and P. Libby (2008), 'Inflammation in atherosclerosis', *Clinical Chemistry*, 54 (1), pp.24–38, pubmed.ncbi. nlm.nih.gov/18160725

10 R. M. Ortega, A. Palencia and A. M. López-Sobaler (2006), 'Improvement of cholesterol levels and reduction of cardiovascular risk via the consumption of phytosterols', *British Journal of Nutrition*, 96 (S1), pp.S89–93, pubmed.ncbi.nlm. nih.gov/16923260; M. B. Katan, S. M. Grundy, P. Jones et al. (2003), 'Efficacy and safety of plant stanols and sterols in the management of blood cholesterol levels', *Mayo Clinic Proceedings*, 78 (8), pp.965–78, pubmed.ncbi.nlm.nih. gov/12911045

11 S. Devries (2017), 'Coronary artery disease: Red yeast rice', in David Rakel (ed.), *Integrative Medicine*, 4th edn (Amsterdam: Elsevier)

12 H. Bader Ul Ain, F. Saeed, M. Tauseef Sultan et al. (2020), 'Effect of thermally treated barley dietary fiber against hypercholesterolemia', *Food Science and Nutrition*, 8 (10), pp.5259–66, pubmed.ncbi.nlm.nih.gov/33133528; H. V. T. Ho, J. L. Sievenpiper, A. Zurbau et al. (2020), 'The effect of oat beta-glucan on LDL-cholesterol,

non-HDL-cholesterol and apoB for CVD risk reduction', *British Journal of Nutrition*, 116 (8), pp.1369–82, pubmed. ncbi.nlm.nih.gov/27724985; X. Zhu, X. Sun, M. Wang et al.(2015), 'Quantitative assessment of the effects of beta-glucan consumption on serum lipid profile and glucose level in hypercholesterolemic subjects', *Nutrition, Metabolism and Cardiovascular Diseases*, 25 (8), pp.714–23, pubmed.ncbi.nlm. nih.gov/26026211

13 P. Hernández-Alonso, J. Salas-Salvadó, M. Baldrich-Mora et al. (2014), 'Beneficial effect of pistachio consumption on glucose metabolism, insulin resistance, inflammation, and related metabolic risk markers', *Diabetes Care*, 37 (11), pp. 3098–105, pubmed.ncbi.nlm.nih.gov/25125505; S. Gulati, A. Misra, R. Mohan Pandey et al. (2014), 'Effects of pistachio nuts on body composition, metabolic, inflammatory and oxidative stress parameters in Asian Indians with metabolic syndrome', *Nutrition*, 30 (2), pp.192–7, pubmed.ncbi. nlm.nih.gov/24377454; J. Salas-Salvadó, M. Bulló, N. Babio et al. (2011), 'Reduction in the incidence of type 2 diabetes with the Mediterranean diet', *Diabetes Care*, 34 (1), pp.14–19, pubmed.ncbi.nlm.nih.gov/20929998; D. J. A. Jenkins, C. W. C. Kendall, A. Marchie et al. (2002), 'Dose response of almonds on coronary heart disease risk factors', *Circulation*, 106 (11), pp.1327–32, pubmed.ncbi.nlm.nih.gov/12221048; V. Mohan, R. Gayathri, L. M. Jaacks et al. (2018), 'Cashew nut consumption increases HDL cholesterol and reduces systolic blood pressure in Asian Indians with type 2 diabetes', *Journal of Nutrition*, 148 (1), pp.63–9, pubmed.ncbi. nlm.nih.gov/29378038

4. Heart Attack and Chest Pain

1 T. Wilbert-Lampen, D. Leistner, S. Greven et al. (2008), 'Cardiovascular events during World Cup soccer', *New England Journal of Medicine*, 358, pp.475–83, doi.org/10.1056/NEJMoa0707427

2 J. S. Hochman, J. E. Tamis, T. D. Thompson et al. (1999), 'Sex, clinical presentation, and outcome in patients with acute coronary symptoms', *New England Journal of Medicine*, 341, pp.266–32, www.nejm.org/doi/10.1056/NEJM199907223410402

3 R. Madsen and R. Birkelune (2016), 'Women's experience during myocardial infarction', *Journal of Clinical Nursing*, 25 (5–6), pp.599–609, pubmed.ncbi.nlm.nih.gov/26771091

4 J. Mehilli and P. Presbitero (2020), 'Coronary artery disease and acute coronary syndrome in women', *Heart*, 106, pp. 487–92, heart.bmj.com/content/106/7/487

5 G. Siasos, V. Tsigkou, E. Kokkou et al. (2014), 'Smoking and atherosclerosis', *Current Medicinal Chemistry*, 21 (34), pp. 3936–48, pubmed.ncbi.nlm.nih.gov/25174928; X. Cheng, E. Ferino, H. Hull et al. (2019), 'Smoking affects gene expression in blood of patients with ischemic stroke', *Annals of Clinical and Translational Neurology*, 6 (9), pp.1748–56, pubmed.ncbi.nlm.nih.gov/31436916

6 I. Gonçalves, E. Andersson Georgiadou, S. Mattsson et al. (2015), 'Direct association with diet and human atherosclerotic plaque', *Scientific Reports*, 5, art.15524, www.nature.com/articles/srep15524

7 M. F. H. Maessen, A. L. M. Verbeek, E. A. Bakker et al. (2016), 'Lifelong exercise patterns and cardiovascular health', *Mayo Clinic Proceedings*, 91 (6), pp.745–54, pubmed.ncbi.nlm.nih.gov/27140541

8 Y. Chang, B.-K. Kim, K. E. Yun et al. (2014), 'Metabolically-healthy obesity and coronary artery calcification', *Journal of the American College of Cardiology*, 63 (24), pp.2679–86, pubmed.ncbi.nlm.nih.gov/24794119; B. Kowall, N. Lehmann, A. A. Mahabadi et al. (2019), 'Associations of metabolically healthy obesity with prevalence and progression of coronary artery calcification', *Nutrition, Metabolism and Cardiovascular Disease*, 29 (3), pp.228–35, pubmed.ncbi.nlm.nih.gov/30648599

9 C. Lassale, I. Tzoulaki, K. G. M. Moons et al. (2018), 'Separate and combined associations of obesity and metabolic health with coronary heart disease', *European Heart Journal*, 39 (5), pp.397–406, pubmed.ncbi.nlm.nih.gov/29020414

10 M.-P. St-Onge, I. Janssen and S. B. Heymsfield (2004), 'Metabolic syndrome in normal-weight Americans', *Diabetes Care*, 27 (9), pp.2222–8, pubmed.ncbi.nlm.nih.gov/15333488

11 Framingham Heart Study, framinghamheartstudy.org/fhs-about

12 U. Wilbert-Lampen, D. Leistner, S. Greven et al. (2008), 'Cardiovascular events during World Cup soccer', *New England Journal of Medicine*, 358, pp.475–83, doi.org/10.1056/NEJMoa0707427

13 M. A. Mohammad, S. Karlsson, J. Haddad et al. (2018), 'Christmas, national holidays, sports events, and time factors as triggers of acute myocardial infarction', *BMJ*, 2018:363: k4811, doi.org/10.1136/bmj.k4811

14 J. Leor, W. K. Poole and R. A. Kloner (1996), 'Sudden cardiac death triggered by an earthquake', *New England Journal of Medicine*, 334, pp.413–19, www.nejm.org/doi/full/10.1056/NEJM199602153340701

15 G. Saposnik, A. Baibergenova, J. Dang and V. Hachinski (2006), 'Does a birthday predispose to vascular events?', *Neurology*, 67 (2), pp.300–4, doi.org/10.1212/01.wnl.0000217915.06544.aa

16 I. M. Carey, S. M. Shah, S. DeWilde et al. (2014), 'Increased risk of acute cardiovascular events after partner bereavement', *JAMA Internal Medicine*, 174 (4), pp.598–605, pubmed.ncbi.nlm.nih.gov/24566983

17 E. Mostofsky, M. Maclure, J. B. Sherwood et al. (2012), 'Risk of acute myocardial infarction after the death of a significant person in one's life', *Circulation*, 125 (3), pp.491–6, pubmed.ncbi.nlm.nih.gov/22230481

18 M. E. Dupre, L. K. George, G. Liu and E. D. Peterson (2015), 'Association between divorce and risks for acute myocardial infarction', *Cardiovascular Quality and Outcomes*, 8, pp.244–51, pubmed.ncbi.nlm.nih.gov/25872508

19 J. Möller, A. Ahlbom, J. Hulting et al. (2001), 'Sexual activity as a trigger of myocardial infarction', *Heart*, 86 (4), pp.387–90, pubmed.ncbi.nlm.nih.gov/11559674

20 M. Kivimaki, J. Pentti, J. E. Ferrie et al. (2018), 'Work stress and risk of death in men and women with and without cardiometabolic disease', *Lancet Diabetes and Endocrinology*, 6, pp.705–13, pubmed.ncbi.nlm.nih.gov/29884468

21 D. R. Witte, D. E. Grobbee, M. L. Bots and A. W. Hoes (2005), 'Excess cardiac mortality on Monday', *European*

Journal of Epidemiology, 20, pp.395–9, europepmc.org/article/med/16080586

22 S. N. Willich, D. Levy, M. B. Rocco et al. (1987), 'Circadian variation in the incidence of sudden cardiac death in the Framingham Heart Study population', *American Journal of Cardiology*, 60 (10), pp.801–6, pubmed.ncbi.nlm.nih.gov/3661393; J. E. Muller, P. H. Stone, Z. G. Turi et al. (1985), 'Circadian variation in the frequency of onset of acute myocardial infarction', *New England Journal of Medicine*, 313 (21), pp.1315–22, pubmed.ncbi.nlm.nih.gov/2865677

23 M. T. Kearney, A. Charlesworth, A. J. Cowley and I. A. Macdonald (2000), 'William Heberden revisited', *Journal of the American College of Cardiology*, 29 (2), pp.302–7, pubmed.ncbi.nlm.nih.gov/9014981

24 X. Wang, Y. Jiang, Y. Bai et al. (2020), 'Association between air temperature and the incidence of acute coronary heart disease in northeast China', *Clinical Interventions in Aging*, 15, pp.47–52, pubmed.ncbi.nlm.nih.gov/8113545

25 T. M. Ikäheimo (2018), 'Cardiovascular diseases, cold exposure and exercise', *Temperature*, 5 (2), pp.123–46, pubmed.ncbi.nlm.nih.gov/30377633

26 A. Putot, F. Chague, P. Manckoundia et al. (2019), 'Post-infectious myocardial infarction', *Journal of Clinical Medicine*, 8 (6), p.827, www.ncbi.nlm.nih.gov/pmc/articles/PMC6616657

27 M. De Hert, J. Detraux and D. Vancampfort (2018), 'The intriguing relationship between coronary heart disease and mental disorders', *Dialogues in Clinical Neuroscience*, 20 (1), pp.31–40, www.ncbi.nlm.nih.gov/pmc/articles/PMC6016051

28 R. Al-Lamee, D. Thompson, H.-M. Dehbi et al. (2018), 'Percutaneous coronary intervention in stable angina

(ORBITA)', *The Lancet*, 391 (10115), pp.31–40, pubmed.
ncbi.nlm.nih.gov/29103656

5. Rhythm Disorders

1 M.-Y. Kim, P. B. Lim, C. Coyle et al. (2020), 'A single ectopy-triggering ganglionated plexus ablation without pulmonary vein isolation prevents atrial fibrillation', *JACC Case Reports*, 2 (12), pp.2004–9, www.jacc.org/doi/full/10.1016/j.jaccas.2020.07.058

2 R. K. Sandhu, J. A. Bakal, J. A. Ezekowitz and F. A. McAlister (2011), 'Risk stratification schemes, anticoagulation use and outcomes', *Heart*, 97 (24), pp.2046–50, heart.bmj.com/content/97/24/2046

3 A. A. Y. Ragab, G. D. S. Sitorus, B. B. J. J. M. Brundel and N. M. S. de Groot (2020), 'The genetic puzzle of familial atrial fibrillation', *Frontiers of Cardiovascular Medicine*, 7, p.14, doi.org/10.3389/fcvm.2020.00014

4 R. Nieuwlaat, A. Capucci, A. J. Camm et al. (2005), 'Atrial fibrillation management', *European Heart Journal*, 26 (22), pp.2422–34, pubmed.ncbi.nlm.nih.gov/16204266

5 P. B. Lim, D. Robb and P. D. Lambiase (2012), 'Electrophysiology and ablation of arrhythmias', *British Journal of Hospital Medicine*, 73 (6), pp.31–8, pubmed.ncbi.nlm.nih.gov/22875320

6 A. Sau, J. P. Howard, S. Al-Aidarous et al. (2019), 'Meta-analysis of randomized controlled trials of atrial fibrillation ablation with pulmonary vein isolation versus without', *JACC Clinical Electrophysiology*, 5 (8), pp.968–76, pubmed.ncbi.nlm.nih.gov/31439299

6. Fainting

1 A. P. Fitzpatrick and P. Cooper (2006), 'Diagnosis and management of patients with blackouts', *Heart*, 92 (4), pp.559–68, www.ncbi.nlm.nih.gov/pmc/articles/PMC1860900

2 R. M. F. L. da Silva (2014), 'Syncope', *Frontiers of Physiology*, 5, p.471, www.ncbi.nlm.nih.gov/pmc/articles/PMC4258989

7. Eating for a Healthy Heart

1 I. Shai, D. Schwarzfuchs, Y. Henkin et al. (2008), 'Weight loss with a low-carbohydrate, Mediterranean, or low-fat diet', *New England Journal of Medicine*, 359, pp.229–41, www.nejm.org/doi/full/10.1056/nejmoa0708681

2 A. Keys (ed.), (1980), *Seven Countries* (Cambridge, MA: Harvard University Press)

3 D. Unwin, D. Haslam and G. Livesey (2016), 'It is the glycaemic response to, not the carbohydrate content of food that matters in diabetes and obesity', *Journal of Insulin Resistance*, 1 (1), art.a8, doi.org/10.4102/jir.v1i1.8

4 H. Ning, D. R. Labarthe, C. M. Shay et al. (2015), 'Status of cardiovascular health in US children up to 11 years of age', *Circulation: Cardiovascular Quality and Outcomes*, 8 (2), pp.164–71, doi.org/10.1161/CIRCOUTCOMES.114.00174

5 Q. Sun, J. Li and F. Gao (2014), 'New insights into insulin', *World Journal of Diabetes*, 5 (2), pp.89–96, www.ncbi.nlm.nih.gov/pmc/articles/PMC3992527

6 K. Naishida and K. Otsu (2017), 'Inflammation and metabolic cardiomyopathy', *Cardiovascular Research*, 113 (4),

pp.389–98, pubmed.ncbi.nlm.nih.gov/28395010; G. Frati, L. Shirone, I. Chimenti et al. (2017), 'An overview of the inflammatory signalling mechanisms in the myocardium underlying the development of diabetic cardiomyopathy', *Cardiovascular Research*, 113 (4), pp.378–88, pubmed.ncbi. nlm.nih.gov/28395009

7 J. H. O'Keefe, N. Torres-Acosta, E. L. O'Keefe et al. (2020), 'A pesco-Mediterranean diet with intermittent fasting', *Journal of the American College of Cardiology*, 76 (12), pp.1484–93, www.jacc.org/doi/full/10.1016/j. jacc.2020.07.049

8 S. Hameed, V. Salem, H. Alessimii et al. (2021), 'Imperial Satiety Protocol', *Diabetes, Obesity and Metabolism*, 23 (1), pp.270–5, doi.org/10.1111/dom.14207

9 R. Lustig (2014), *Fat Chance* (London: Fourth Estate)

10 C. B. Esselstyn Jr. (2007), *Prevent and Reverse Heart Disease* (New York: Avery)

11 Interview with Bill Clinton (2010), *The Situation Room*, CNN, 24 September 2010, transcripts.cnn.com/TRAN-SCRIPTS/1009/24/sitroom.02.html

12 D. Buettner, *The Blue Zones*, 2nd edn (Washington, DC: National Geographic Books)

13 E. R. Ropelle, M. B. Flores, D. E. Cintra et al. (2010), 'IL-6 and IL-10 anti-inflammatory activity links exercise to hypo-thalamic insulin and leptin sensitivity through IKKß and ER stress inhibition', *PLoS Biology*, 8 (8), art.e1000465, www. ncbi.nlm.nih.gov/pmc/articles/PMC2927536

14 T. J. Hatton (2014), 'How have Europeans grown so tall?', *Oxford Economic Papers*, 66 (2), pp.349–72, doi.org/10.1093/ oep/gpt030

15 J. E. Cecil, R. Tavendale, P. Watt et al. (2008), 'An obesity-associated *FTO* gene variant and increased energy intake in children', *New England Journal of Medicine*, 359, pp.2558–66, doi.org/10.1056/NEJMoa0803839

16 S. E. Berry, A. M. Valdes, D. A. Drew et al. (2020), 'Human postprandial responses to food and potential for precision nutrition', *Nature Medicine*, 26 (6), pp.964–73, pubmed.ncbi.nlm.nih.gov/32528151

8. Exercising for a Stronger Heart

1 M. J. Joyner and D. J. Green (2009), 'Exercise protects the cardiovascular system', *Journal of Physiology*, 587 (23), pp.5551–8, pubmed.ncbi.nlm.nih.gov/19736305

2 K. M. Beavers, T. E. Brinkley and B. J. Nicklas (2010), 'Effect of exercise training on chronic inflammation', *Clinica Chimica Acta: International Journal of Clinical Chemistry*, 411 (0), pp.785–93, www.ncbi.nlm.nih.gov/pmc/articles/PMC3629815

3 B. K. Pedersen and B. Saltin (2015), 'Exercise as medicine', *Scandinavian Journal of Medicine & Science in Sports*, 25 (3), pp.1–72, https://pubmed.ncbi.nlm.nih.gov/26606383/

4 Ibid.

5 H. B. Simon (2015), 'Exercise and health', *American Journal of Medicine*, 128 (11), pp.1171–7, doi.org/10.1016/j.amjmed.2015.05.012

6 I.-M. Lee, E. J. Shiroma, M. Kamada et al. (2019), 'Association of step volume and intensity with all-cause mortality in older women', *JAMA Internal Medicine*, 179 (9), pp.1105–12, doi.org/jamainternmed.2019.0899

7 J. Helgerud, K. Høydal, E. Wang et al. (2007), 'Aerobic high-intensity intervals improve VO2max more than moderate training', *Medicine and Science in Sports and Exercise*, 39 (4), pp.665–71, pubmed.ncbi.nlm.nih.gov/17414804

8 Q. Fu and B. D. Levine (2013), 'Exercise and the autonomic nervous system', *Handbook of Clinical Neurology*, 117, pp.147–60, pubmed.ncbi.nlm.nih.gov/24095123

9 J. A. Blumenthal, M. Fredrikson, C. M. Kuhn et al. (1990), 'Aerobic exercise reduces levels of cardiovascular and sympathoadrenal responses to mental stress in subjects without prior evidence of myocardial ischemia', *American Journal of Cardiology*, 65 (1), pp.93–8, pubmed.ncbi.nlm.nih.gov/2294687

9. Creating a Better Balance between Stress and Rest

1 J. M. Da Costa (1871; reprinted 1951), 'On irritable heart', *American Journal of Medicine*, 11 (5), pp.559–67, doi.org/10.1016/0002-9343(51)90038-1

2 M. Dani, A. Dirksen, P. Taraborrelli et al. (2020), 'Autonomic dysfunction in "long COVID"', *Clinical Medicine* (pre-print 26 November 2020), pubmed.ncbi.nlm.nih.gov/33243837

3 T. H. Sato, T. Uchida, K. Dote and M. Ishihara (1990), 'Tako-tsubo-like left ventricular dysfunction due to multivessel coronary spasm', in K. Kodama, K. Haze and M. Hori (eds), *Clinical Aspect of Myocardial Injury* (Tokyo: Kagaku Hyoron-sha Publishing), pp.56–64

4 H. Paur, P. T. Wright, M. B. Sikkel et al. (2012), High levels of circulating epinephrine trigger apical cardiodepression',

Circulation, 126, pp.697–706, pubmed.ncbi.nlm.nih.gov/22732314

5 P. Eshtehardi, S. C. Koestner, P. Adorjan et al. (2009), 'Transient apical ballooning syndrome', *International Journal of Cardiology*, 135 (3), pp.370–5, pubmed.ncbi.nlm.nih.gov/18599137

6 H. F. J. González, A. Yengo-Kahn and D. J. Englot (2019), 'Vagus nerve stimulation for the treatment of epilepsy', *Neurosurgery Clinics of North America*, 30 (2), pp.219–30, pubmed.ncbi.nlm.nih.gov/30898273; I. S. Anand, M. A. Konstam, H. U. Klein et al. (2020), 'Comparison of symptomatic and functional responses to vagus nerve stimulation in ANTHEM-HF, INOVATE-HF, and NECTAR-HF', *European Journal of Heart Failure*, 7 (1), pp.75–83, pubmed.ncbi.nlm.nih.gov/31984682; J. Hadaya and J. L. Ardell (2020), 'Autonomic modulation for cardiovascular disease', *Frontiers in Physiology*, 11, art.617459, www.ncbi.nlm.nih.gov/pmc/articles/PMC7783451

7 S. W. Porges (2011), 'The polyvagal theory: New insights into adaptive reactions of the autonomic nervous system', *Cleveland Clinic Journal of Medicine*, 76 (S2), pp.S86–90, www.ncbi.nlm.nih.gov/pmc/articles/PMC3108032; M. B. Sullivan, M. Erb, L. Schmalzl et al. (2018), 'Yoga therapy and polyvagal theory', *Frontiers in Human Neuroscience*, 12, p.67, www.ncbi.nlm.nih.gov/pmc/articles/PMC5835127

8 A. Gill Taylor, L. E. Goehler, D. I. Galper et al. (2010), 'Top-down and bottom-up mechanisms in mind-body medicine', *Explore*, 6 (1), pp.29–41, pubmed.ncbi.nlm.nih.gov/20129310

9 T. Brosse (1946), 'A psycho-physiological study', *Main Currents in Modern Thought*, 4, p.77; W. Broad (2013), *The Science of Yoga* (New York: Simon & Schuster); J. Hamblin (2014), 'Dead or meditating?', *Atlantic*, 30 May 2014, www.theatlantic. com/health/archive/2014/05/dead-or-meditating/371846

10 S. Overhaus, H. Rüddel, I. Curio et al. (2003), 'Biofeedback of baroreflex sensitivity in patients with mild essential hypertension', *International Journal of Behavioral Medicine*, 10 (1), pp.66–78, www.ncbi.nlm.nih.gov/pubmed/12581949; J. M. Del Pozo, R. N. Gevirtz, B. Scher and E. Guarneri (2004), 'Biofeedback treatment increases heart rate variability in patients with known coronary artery disease', *American Heart Journal*, 147 (3), p.545, doi.org/10.1016/j. ahj.2003.08.013; F. Luskin, M. Reitz, K. Newell et al. (2002), 'A controlled pilot study of stress management training of elderly patients with congestive heart failure', *Preventive Cardiology*, 5 (4), pp.168–74, pubmed.ncbi.nlm.nih.gov/12417824

11 R. H. Schneider, C. E. Grim, M. V. Rainforth et al. (2012), 'Stress reduction in the secondary prevention of cardiovascular disease', *Circulation, Cardiovascular Quality and Outcomes*, 5 (6), pp.750–8, pubmed.ncbi.nlm.nih.gov/23149426

12 L. Besedovsky, T. Lange and J. Born (2012), 'Sleep and immune function', *European Journal of Physiology*, 463, pp.121–37, link.springer.com/article/10.1007/s00424-011-1044-0

13 O. Tochikubo, A. Ikeda, E. Miyajima and M. Ishii (1996), 'Effects of insufficient sleep on blood pressure monitored by a new multibiomedical recorder', *Hypertension*, 27 (6), pp.1318–24, pubmed.ncbi.nlm.nih.gov/8641742

14 F. P. Cappuccio, D. Cooper, L. D'Elia et al. (2011), 'Sleep duration predicts cardiovascular outcomes', *European Heart Journal*, 32 (12), pp.1484–92, pubmed.ncbi.nlm.nih.gov/21300732

15 M. Walker (2018), *Why We Sleep* (London: Penguin)

16 K. L. Knutson and E. Van Cauter (2015), 'Associations between sleep loss and increased risk of obesity and diabetes', *Annals of the New York Academy of Sciences*, 1129, pp.287–304, www.ncbi.nlm.nih.gov/pmc/articles/PMC4394987

17 M. Nollet, W. Wisden and N. P. Franks (2020), 'Sleep deprivation and stress', *Interface Focus*, 10 (3), 20190092, pubmed.ncbi.nlm.nih.gov/32382403

18 N. Rafique, L. Ibrahim Al-Asoom, A. Abdulrahman Alsunni et al. (2020), 'Effects of mobile use on subjective sleep quality', *Nature and Science of Sleep*, 12, pp.357–64, www.ncbi.nlm.nih.gov/pmc/articles/PMC7320888

19 R. A. Bryant (2016), 'Social attachments and traumatic stress', *European Journal of Psychotraumatology*, 7, art.29065, www.ncbi.nlm.nih.gov/pmc/articles/PMC4800287

20 X. Lu, H.-S. Juon, X. He et al. (2019), 'The association between perceived stress and hypertension among Asian Americans', *Journal of Community Health*, 44 (3), pp.451–62, www.ncbi.nlm.nih.gov/pmc/articles/PMC6504578

21 K. Orth-Gomér, A. Rosengren and L. Wilhelmsen (1993), 'Lack of social support and incidence of coronary heart disease in middle-aged Swedish men', *Psychosomatic Medicine*, 55 (1), pp.37–43, pubmed.ncbi.nlm.nih.gov/8446739

22 J. Abel, H. Kingston, A. Scally et al. (2018), 'Reducing emergency hospital admissions', *British Journal of General Practice*, 68 (676), pp.e803–10, doi.org/10.3399/bjgp18X699437

23 S. E. Taylor (2006), 'Tend and befriend', *Current Directions in Psychological Science*, 15 (6), pp.273–7, doi.org/10.1111/j.1467-8721.2006.00451.x

24 L. Jans-Beken, N. Jacobs, M. Janssens et al. (2020), 'Gratitude and health', *Journal of Positive Psychology*, 15 (6), pp.743–82, doi.org/10.1080/17439760.2019.1651888

25 E. A. Locke and G. P. Latham (2006), 'New directions in goal-setting theory', *Current Directions in Psychological Science*, 15 (5), pp.265–8, doi.org/10.1111/j.1467-8721.2006.00449.x

26 G. Matthews (2015), 'Goals research summary', quoted in Sarah Gardner and Dave Albee, 'Study focuses on strategies for achieving goals, resolutions', Dominican University of California, 1 February 2015, scholar.dominican.edu/cgi/viewcontent.cgi?article=1265&context=news-releases

10. Caring for Your Heart, Holistically

1 C. M. DuBois, O. Vesga Lopez, E. E. Beale et al. (2015), 'Relationships between positive psychological constructs and health outcomes in patients with cardiovascular disease', *International Journal of Cardiology*, 195, pp.265–80, pubmed.ncbi.nlm.nih.gov/26048390

2 N. M. Radcliffe and W. M. P. Klein (2002), 'Dispositional, unrealistic and comparative optimism', *Personality and Social Psychology Bulletin*, 28 (6), pp.836–46, doi.org/10.1177/0146167202289012

3 L. Solberg Nes and S. C. Segerstrom (2006), 'Dispositional optimism and coping', *Personality and Social Psychology Review*, 10 (3), pp.235–51, pubmed.ncbi.nlm.nih.gov/16859439

4 L. Brydon, C. Walker, A. J. Wawrzyniak et al. (2009), 'Dispositional optimism and stress-induced changes in immunity and negative mood', *Brain, Behavior, and Immunity*, 23 (6), pp.810–16, www.ncbi.nlm.nih.gov/pmc/articles/PMC2715885

5 A. Huffington (2019), 'Microsteps', Thrive Global, thriveglobal.com/stories/microsteps-big-idea-too-small-to-fail-healthy-habits-willpower

6 M. Muraven, R. F. Baumeister and D. M. Tice (1999), 'Longitudinal improvement of self-regulation through practice', *Journal of Social Psychology*, 139 (4), pp.446–57, pubmed.ncbi.nlm.nih.gov/10457761

Further Reading and Resources

On my website, drboonlim.co.uk/heart-healthy, you will find useful videos illustrating pulse checks, blood-pressure measurements, breathing exercises and the heart in action, as well as blogs about new developments in the medical treatment of some heart problems.

I also find the following resources useful when talking with people about building and committing to lifestyle changes that will make their heart healthier.

Monitoring your blood pressure

Stride BP, stridebp.org/bp-monitors. A list of preferred and scientifically validated blood-pressure monitors for use at home

Understanding your risk of heart attack or stroke

MD Calc Framingham Risk Score for Hard Coronary Heart Disease, www.mdcalc.com/framingham-risk-score-hard-coronary-heart-disease

MD Calc Reynolds Risk Score for Cardiovascular Risk in Women, www.mdcalc.com/reynolds-risk-score-cardiovascular-risk-women

QRISK®3-2018 calculator, qrisk.org/three/index.php. My preferred risk calculator, because it allows you to play around with a range of inputs to see how lifestyle changes can improve your risk profile

Stopping fainting

Stop Fainting, www.stopfainting.com. Tips for reducing the frequency of blackouts (syncope) due to low blood pressure

Stopping smoking

NHS stop-smoking services, www.nhs.uk/live-well/quit-smoking/nhs-stop-smoking-services-help-you-quit

US Centers for Disease Control (CDC) Tobacco Control Programs, www.cdc.gov/tobacco/stateand-community/tobacco_control_programs/index.htm. A map that enables people to locate stop-smoking services in their community

Eating more healthfully

Dan Buettner (2012), *The Blue Zones: 9 Lessons for Living Longer from the People Who've Lived the Longest*, 2nd edn (Washington, DC: National Geographic Books)

Jason Fung (2016), *The Obesity Code: Unlocking the Secrets of Weight Loss* (London: Scribe)

Robert Lustig (2014), *Fat Chance: The Hidden Truth about Sugar, Obesity and Disease* (London: Fourth Estate)

Satchin Panda (2018), *The Circadian Code: Lose Weight, Supercharge Your Energy and Sleep Well Every Night* (London: Vermilion)

Tim Spector (2020), *Spoon-Fed: Why Almost Everything We've Been Told about Food is Wrong* (London: Jonathan Cape)

London Metabolic Clinic, www.londonmetaboliclaboratory. com. A clinic focused on developing personalized nutrition programmes through continuous blood-glucose monitoring, offering services to people globally

NHS BMI healthy weight calculator, www.nhs.uk/live-well/ healthy-weight/bmi-calculator

University of Sydney, Boden Institute of Obesity, Nutrition, Exercise & Eating Disorders Glycemic Index, www.glycemic-index.com

Exercising more regularly

Daniel Lieberman (2020), *Exercised: The Science of Physical Activity, Rest and Health* (London: Allen Lane)

MapMyWalk, www.mapmywalk.com. Step and mileage tracking app for smartphones

Nitric Oxide Dump workout, www.nitricoxidedump.com. Dr Zach Bush's four-minute high-intensity interval training (HIIT) workout

Strava, www.strava.com. Step and mileage tracking app for smartphones

Managing stress more effectively

Héctor Garcia and Francesc Miralles (2017), *Ikigai: The Japanese Secret to a Long and Happy Life* (London: Hutchinson)

Wim Hof (2020), *The Wim Hof Method: Activate Your Potential, Transcend Your Limits* (London: Rider)

Jon Kabat-Zinn (2013), *Full Catastrophe Living: How to Cope with Stress, Pain and Illness Using Mindfulness Meditation*, rev. edn (London: Piatkus)

James Nestor (2020), *Breath: The New Science of a Lost Art* (London: Penguin Life)

Mark Williams and Danny Penman (2011), *Mindfulness: A Practical Guide to Finding Peace in a Frantic World* (London: Piatkus). Includes CD with guided meditations

Calm app, www.calm.com. Mindfulness meditation app for smartphones

Headspace app, www.headspace.com. Mindfulness meditation app for smartphones

HeartMath, www.heartmath.com. Training and devices that nurture a stronger awareness of heart health and help to improve stress responses (use the code STOPFAINT-ING10 for a 10 per cent discount on products)

POTS UK, www.potsuk.org. An organization dedicated to increasing awareness and support for people with postural orthostatic tachycardia syndrome

Caring for your heart, holistically

Arianna Huffington (2019), 'Microsteps: The big idea that's too small to fail', Thrive Global, thriveglobal.com/stories/microsteps-big-idea-too-small-to-fail-healthy-habits-willpower

Daniel Levitin (2020), *The Changing Mind: A Neuroscientist's Guide to Ageing Well* (London: Penguin Life)

Feel Better, Live More podcast from Dr Rangan Chatterjee, drchatterjee.com/blog/category/podcast

PositivePsychology.com, tools.positivepsychology.com/ebook. Positive psychology exercises from Martin Seligman

Learning more about heart conditions

Many countries have national heart foundations or associations that provide a range of education, research and support.

American Heart Association, www.heart.org. The main education, research and support charity in the US for heart health, it has information for patients and organizes online and local support groups (supportnetwork.heart.org)

British Heart Foundation, www.bhf.org.uk. The main education, research and support charity in the UK for heart health, it has information for patients and organizes online and local support groups (www.bhf.org.uk/informationsupport/support/heart-support-groups)

Heart Foundation (Australia), www.heartfoundation.org.au. The main education, research and support charity in Australia for heart health

Heart & Stroke (Canada), www.heartandstroke.ca. The main education, research and support charity in Canada for heart health

Amit V. Khera, Connor A. Emdin, Isabel Drake et al. (2016), 'Genetic risk, adherence to a healthy lifestyle, and coronary disease', *New England Journal of Medicine*, 375 (24), pp.2349–58, pubmed.ncbi.nlm.nih.gov/27959714

Living with a heart condition

If you have been diagnosed with a heart problem, your doctors or hospital will be able to suggest local support groups. Many offer nutrition, exercise and stress-management programmes for patients, some of which may be tailored specifically to people with heart problems and are free. Ask your team to signpost programmes available in your area.

Arrhythmia Alliance UK, www.heartrhythmalliance.org/aa/uk. UK charity for people with heart-rhythm disorders. It is a member of the global Arrhythmia Alliance, which has organizations in twenty-seven countries. These can be found through the Arrhythmia Alliance portal at www.heartrhythm alliance.org

Cardiomyopathy UK, www.cardiomyopathy.org. UK charity for people with weakened heart muscles and other heart-muscle problems

Chest, Heart & Stroke Scotland, www.chss.org.uk. Scotland's main charity for people with cardiovascular conditions

Heart UK, www.heartuk.org.uk. UK charity for people with cholesterol problems

Syncope Trust And Reflex anoxic Seizures (STARS), www.heartrhythmalliance.org/stars/uk. UK charity for people with vasovagal and other types of syncope

WomenHeart, www.womenheart.org. US charity for women with, or at risk of, heart problems

Acknowledgements

I have many people to be grateful to.

To my father, who is my greatest inspiration – much of who I am today has been directly shaped by you. To my mother, for her unconditional love and unbridled zest for life.

To my wife, Wei Li, who has put up with the many lost weekends and has supported me throughout. To my children, Ethan and Emily, who continue to teach me far more than I could teach them.

To my brothers, Wu and Jin, for their perseverance in educating me in life's greater purpose.

I am grateful to Dr Ramzi Khamis and Dr Saira Hameed, who have helped me with specific chapters of this book. To my family within the Imperial Syncope Group, including Trish, Andreas, Mel, Miriam and my mentor Professor Richard Sutton, who continue to inspire me to be better. To Simi and Debbie, who have always got my back. To all my wonderful and supportive colleagues at Imperial, particularly Professor Prapa Kanagaratnam, for his unwavering guidance over the years.

I am grateful to Lydia Yadi, my editor at Penguin, and the rest of the team at Penguin Random House for giving me the opportunity to write this book. And to Robin Dennis, a phenomenal editor, who helped me crystallize some technical concepts over early mornings, weekends and holidays, graciously fitting herself into my schedule.

ACKNOWLEDGEMENTS

To every single one of my patients, who have inspired me to live by one of my favourite mottos: to learn something new every day.

And, finally, I'm immensely grateful that you have decided to read this book. My deep hope is that it helps you unlock healing on your journey into heart health.

PREPARING FOR THE PERIMENOPAUSE AND MENOPAUSE

DR LOUISE NEWSON

Part of the Penguin Life Experts series.

Dr Louise Newson is the UK's leading menopause specialist, and she's determined to help women thrive during the menopause.

Despite being something that almost every woman will experience at some point in their lives, menopause is frequently misdiagnosed and misinformation and stigma are commonplace. Dr Newson demystifies the menopause and explains why every woman should be perimenopause-aware, regardless of their age.

Using new research, expert advice and empowering patient stories from a diverse range of women who have struggled to secure adequate treatment and correct diagnosis, Dr Newson equips readers with expert advice and practical tips. She empowers women to confidently take charge of their health and their changing bodies.

It's never too early to learn about the perimenopause or menopause and this compact guide will provide you with everything you need to know.